ANXIETY DISORDERS - FROM CHILDHOOD TO ADULTHOOD

Edited by **Neşe Kocabaşoğlu**
and **R. Hülya Bingöl Çağlayan**

Anxiety Disorders - From Childhood to Adulthood
http://dx.doi.org/10.5772/intechopen.74272
Edited by Neşe Kocabaşoğlu and R. Hülya Bingöl Çağlayan

Contributors

Fugen Neziroglu, Luis Pando-Orellana, Kentaro Shirotsuki, Shota Noda, Daniel Guerra, Gokcen Akyurek, Kübra Sahadet Sezer, Leyla Kaya, Keziban Temuçin, Irene Minja, Febronia Kahabuka, Hulya Bingol Caglayan

Notice

First published in London, United Kingdom, 2019 by IntechOpen
IntechOpen is the global imprint of INTECHOPEN LIMITED, registered in England and Wales, registration number: 11086078, The Shard, 25th floor, 32 London Bridge Street
London, SE19SG – United Kingdom
Printed in Croatia

British Library Cataloguing-in-Publication Data
A catalogue record for this book is available from the British Library

Additional hard copies can be obtained from orders@intechopen.com

Anxiety Disorders - From Childhood to Adulthood, Edited by Neşe Kocabaşoğlu and R. Hülya Bingöl Çağlayan
p. cm.
Print ISBN 978-1-78985-481-7
Online ISBN 978-1-78985-482-4

Meet the editors

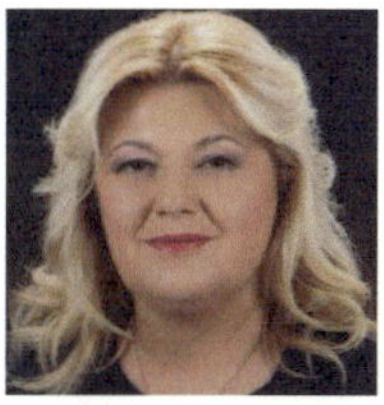

Professor Doctor Neşe Kocabaşoğlu was born in 1960 in Istanbul, Turkey. She graduated from Besiktas Ataturk Deneme High School in 1977 and from Istanbul University Cerrahpasa Medical Faculty in 1983. She completed her mandatory medical service in Mersin, Turkey from 1984 to 1986. In 1986, she returned to Cerrahpasa Medical Faculty and started as an assistant doctor in the Psychiatry Department. When she became a psychiatry specialist in 1991, she started to work as a teaching assistant in the same department. In 1995, she received the title of associate professor. She became a professor in 2001 and is still a professor lecturer at the Cerrahpasa Medical Faculty. She is a founder member of the Turkish Psychiatry Association, founded in 1995 and has its headquarters in Ankara. She is also a member of the Sexual Health Institute (CİSED) in Turkey and an international member of the American Psychiatry Association. She works as the publishing secretary of the regularly published magazines New Symposium Psychiatry and Neurological Sciences Magazine as well as a publishing advisory committee member of the Okmeydani Medical Journal and Clinical Psychopharmalogical Journal. She has undertaken a large amount of research on social psychiatry and anxiety disorders. Parallel to her work, she founded the Cerrahpasa Medical Faculty Psychiatry Department's Anxiety Disorders Unit. Since 2002, she has been working as the commission member of the Ministry of Justice Forensic Medicine Institution's Observation Specialization Department. She obtained the first-place award for psychiatric research in 39. National Psychiatry Congress with her work "Late Beginning in Post-Traumatic Stress Disorder and Investigation of Factors Related to Chronic Illness". Her national and international research has been published in over 200 sources and she is currently working on multiple ongoing research. She can speak Turkish and English, is married and has a daughter.

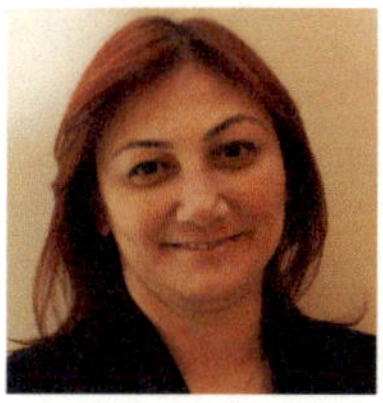

R. Hülya Bingöl Çağlayan graduated from the Private Tarhan College in 1990. In 1997, she graduated from the English program at the Cerrahpaşa Faculty of Medicine. From 1999 to 2001, she worked as an Assistant Doctor to Prof. Dr. H. Przuntek at the Germany Ruhr University Neurology Clinic and worked in the Chorea Huntington Center. Later, she completed her specialization in LWL Klinik Marl-Sinsen, *Haardklinik*, at the Germany hospital, in a specialized region hospital as a Child and Adolescent Psychiatrist and Psychotherapist. She completed the adult psychiatry residency in LWL-Universitätsklinikum in Bochum by Prof. Dr. Georg Juckel. She returned to Turkey in 2008 and since then, she has been working at the Istanbul University Cerrahpaşa School of Medicine as a specialist in the Department of Child and Adolescent Psychiatry Clinic.

She is specialized in cognitive behavioral therapies and psychodrama from her years as a specialist in Germany and qualified to be a child and adolescent psychotherapist. From 2012 to 2015, the Ministry of Family and Social Policies requested R. Hülya Bingöl Çağlayan to develop the Divorce Process Consultancy Project, prepare a concept book called Divorce Counseling within the scope of the project and provide the 280 personnel affiliated to the Ministry with special training.
She is still actively providing scientific consultancy for the Istanbul Autism Technical Board in the framework of the National Autism Action Plan.

Contents

Preface

We currently have relatively less information about the mechanisms that contribute to the persistence or recurrence of anxiety across development. Much less diagnostic specificity is evident on the findings in the course of development. Retrospective studies point to the persistence of early anxiety disorders and suggest a relatively chronic or recurrent course. Onset of first anxiety disorder is often followed by the development of other anxieties in adolescence or early adulthood and in its turn, this anxiety predicts other adverse outcomes including depression, substance use, and suicidality along with psychosocial difficulties and poor functioning [1].

In this book, we emphasize the intercourse of different anxiety disorders and underlying mechanisms in a lifetime. Important anxiety disorders such as dental anxiety in children and neurological conditions such as temporal lobe epilepsy are included.

We believe this book will appeal to a wide audience of practicing psychiatrists, psychologists, psychiatric nurses, social workers, and mental health professionals. It is our hope that many will find this book useful for training mental health professionals to give them the newest developmental point of view about prototype anxiety disorders.

We dedicate this book to our lovely families, patients, and their families.

Prof. Dr. Neşe Kocabaşoğlu
İstanbul University-Cerrahpasa
Cerrahpasa School of Medicine
Adult Psychiatry Clinic, Turkey

Dr. R. Hülya Bingöl Çağlayan
İstanbul University-Cerrahpasa
Cerrahpasa School of Medicine
Child and Adolescent Psychiatry Clinic, Turkey

References

[1] Copeland, WE et al. (2014) Longitudinal patterns of anxiety from childhood to adulthood: The Great Smoky Mountains Study.Journal of the American Academy of Child and Adolescent Psychiatry 53, 21-33.

Section 1

Introduction

Chapter 1

Introductory Chapter: Anxiety Disorders and the Precursors

Nese Kocabasoğlu and R. Hülya Bingöl Çağlayan

Additional information is available at the end of the chapter

http://dx.doi.org/10.5772/intechopen.82737

1. Introduction

In the first ideas of this book, we were much concerned about the children with an anxiety disorder and the children whose parents were diagnosed with any anxiety disorders in their lifetime. So, we are eager to check out the different types of anxiety disorders with different underlying mechanisms.

Different anxiety disorders stand out in the center of many psychiatric conditions, independent of developmental periods and age. Accordingly, different anxiety issues play an important role in the psychopathology of a child and adolescent development. Today, we can detect childhood fears earlier and evaluate them as the pioneer of many adult psychiatric disorders.

Epidemiological studies on child and adolescent psychopathology have been conducted since the 1980s. Especially, studies on childhood anxiety are the most common. In this way, risk factors are better determined, leading symptoms are recognized and accordingly prevented, and therapeutic strategies are developed.

The developmental perspective will support a better understanding of the development of anxiety disorders and transition from childhood to adulthood. Developmental psychopathology is concerned with the causes and prognosis of improper misconduct and examines normal and pathological behaviors in the perspective of development. Its predecessors are Thomas Achenbach, Dante Cicchetti, Michael Rutter, and Alan Sroufe.

Each developmental period has its own developmental tasks. As Robert Havighurst described in 1948, development is a lifelong process and different life duties must be fulfilled in each life period [1]. In the meantime, the child is considered as an active learner in continuous communication with his environment. Successful completion of these developmental tasks will ensure that the child and the adolescent maintain their mental health in a healthy way. If these tasks are not fulfilled, it will lead to loss of happiness, loss of success, exclusion by society, and consequently loss of other related development tasks.

Anxiety formation can be understood as the fulfillment of developmental tasks in this background in a way that is not appropriate for the development period. For example, the development of separation anxiety is facilitated if the autonomy development, which is the assignment of the age of 3, is not successful.

An important developmental task of childhood is emotion control. Strategies used in emotion control of children are important in understanding clinical anxiety disorders.

1.1. Development of anxiety emotion

An important discussion in developmental psychology is related to the development of emotions. Does the newborn bring with them feelings or do emotions vary later? Walters and Sroufe [2] argue that emotions will be varied during ontogenesis. The sense of fear develops through steps. It has a sense of not receiving pleasure and is closely related to the child's cognitive and social development. The first observed fear predecessors in the newborn are compulsory attention and insecurity. Fear is activated when there is a negative movement for the child. Izard and Sroufe acknowledge that the first fear appeared in the 7th month. The baby becomes restless if visual stimuli are given to the baby for 10–15 days. First, he reacts calmly and then becomes active, crying and shouting, because the child's activity ability was cut by the object. The content of the visual stimulus is not important here. Infants become restless as a result of a person looking at the baby's face for 30 s. Here, the baby acquainted with other foreign factors. The content of the warning has gained importance. 30 s after the response is the development of fear. In contrast, fear and anxiety arise as a result of stimuli considered threatening.

From the 6th month, if a foreign person suddenly gets in the lap of the child, the babies react. This reaction is observed especially in all infants aged 10–12 months. Here, the foreign person is perceived as a kind of reverse event and creates a negative scheme in infants. This is the pioneer of fear/anxiety. As the age progresses, the content of the stimulus plays a greater role, and the fear is varied and defines this period as mistrust.

Fears are common in childhood. Their contents vary by age and are temporary. The cognitive development and developmental period of the child are in relation. For example, at the end of the first year, they fear foreign people, foreign places, and loud voices. At the age of 4, the fear of darkness, fears of animals, and fears of being left alone come to the surface.

1.2. The risk factors of anxiety development

The most commonly used model in explaining the causes of psychiatric disorders is the diathesis-stress model [3]. Diathesis refers to the Greek predisposition and is considered to be the susceptibility of the individual to both structural and environmental factors and diseases and non-normative behaviors. The definition of an individual's response to any stress caused by the environment can also be extended. This individual predisposition may be determined as genetic, organic, biochemical, psychiatric, and/or social. The concept of diathesis was first used in schizophrenia research [4]. The other definition mentioned with diathesis is the concept of risk.

Risk is defined as the probability of developing an individual's disease within a certain period of time.

Kraemer et al. [5] identified different risk factors. The first step is whether the risk related to the disease occurs concurrently with the disease. Risk factors that are spontaneous or can be changed as a result of any intervention are defined as variable risk factors.

1.2.1. Family as a risk factor

In family research, the incidence of the same disorder is screened in the relatives of people with psychiatric disorders. A number of family studies reported that panic disorder showed familial frequency [21, 22]. In recent years, the subject is frequently investigated and the relationship between the anxiety of children and the anxiety of parents [6, 7].

In the last family researches conducted by Cynthia Last, [8] 83% of the children diagnosed with separation anxiety were found to meet the anxiety disorder criteria at their mothers' lifetime.

About 57% meet the criteria of an anxiety disorder at the time of research. The second major study by Last [9]. Relatives of children with anxiety disorders, relatives of children with attention deficit hyperactivity disorder, and relatives of children without any psychiatric diagnosis were included in the study. Anxiety disorder was found in 40.4% of the parents of children with anxiety disorders. In the other two groups, anxiety disorder was quite low. The most common type of anxiety disorder among children with anxiety disorders is excessive anxiety (18.9%) and phobic disorder (11.7%). Panic disorder, social phobia, obsessive compulsive disorder, and avoidant personality disorders are more common in the relatives of children with anxiety disorders than in the control group.

Children with a diagnosis of anxiety disorder in their parents have a higher risk of developing anxiety disorder. Both axis studies indicate familial clustering in anxiety disorders. Evidence of more specific transitions, especially in panic disorder and social phobia, was obtained.

1.2.2. Biological risk factors

The effect of biological risk factors on the development of childhood and adolescent anxiety disorders was investigated in few studies. Studies on the subject were mostly conducted using adult subjects. In these studies, locus ceruleus, sympathetic system, and HPA axis were investigated. It has been shown that the levels of cortisol increases in the stress of normal children [10]. In studies with children with social anxiety, it was observed that heart rate increased compared to normal children. Kagan [11] found the low stimulus threshold with the participation of the amygdala and hypothalamus in the limbic system in children with anxiety.

Shaffer et al. [12] argued that some of the signals could be interpreted as an anxiety disorder precursor. The parents of children with agora phobia were found to be more frequent than the children who had motor-mild symptoms without the agoraphobia (Kaplan et al. [13]).

1.2.2.1. *Increased startle reaction*

The startle reaction was observed for 6 months from the newborn period (Balaban [14]). In many studies, an increased startle reaction was found in individuals with anxiety disorder compared to the control group [23, 26]. Grillon found that parents with alcohol dependence showed an increased startle reaction to alcohol-dependent parents compared to their children. In the second study performed by the same study group, the startle reaction potentials of the parents of children with different anxiety disorders and the children of parents without a psychiatric disorder were compared. Higher startle potential was determined in girls. As a result, increased startle reaction may be considered as a predisposition factor in the development of anxiety disorder.

1.2.3. *Gender*

Childhood anxiety disorders constitute a risk factor for gender development in girls. Phobic disorder, anxiety disorder, and post-traumatic stress disorder are frequently seen. On the other hand, childhood obsessive compositional disorder is more common in boys. Separation anxiety disorders are seen equally in both sexes [25]. Biological and psychosocial study hypotheses were used to explain gender differences in anxiety disorders. The effects of sex hormones on monthly onset, menopause, pregnancy, and postpartum period anxiety symptoms in biological theories were investigated. In general, these explanations are not sufficient to explain the gender differences that we have found in childhood. Genetic factors are discussed as the cause of anxiety disorders in girls. For example, according to Drowe et al. (1983), the panic disorder is genetically inherited, and the genes responsible for panic disorders in women show a high transition. According to [24], genetic factors play an important role rather than gender-aware environmental factors. At present, it is unclear which gene causes gender difference in anxiety disorders.

1.2.4. *Behavioral inhibition*

Examining the temperament characteristics as the precursors of psychiatric disorders has been an important step in etiology research. The event mentioned as temperament and structurally inherited is defined as the predisposition that determines how the individual behaves against particular people in certain situations. It emerges in the very early period, remains constant at all times, and is influenced by biological factors. Behavioral inhibition is a temperament characteristic.

Behavioral inhibition is defined as avoiding shy, conducting behaviors in the newly entered environment or against newcomers (Kagan [11]). This behavior can be observed from the 8th month. Inhibition of behavior during infancy shows as a disgrace (crying, yelling), as shy and anxious behavior in a small childhood, and as a social recessive behavior in school age. The constancy of this temperament property has been proven in many studies until adulthood (Biederman et al. [12]; Gest [13]; Matheny [14]).

Children with behavioral inhibition according to Kagan show a low stimulation threshold in the amygdala and the hypothalamus, in particular, against foreign conditions. In addition, increased sympathetic stimulation was observed.

According to Kagan the children of individuals with panic disorder and agoraphobia showed more behavioral inhibition than healthy parents (Rosenbaum et al. [15, 16]). According to the results of two prospective studies, children with behavioral inhibition are in a high-risk group in terms of developing childhood anxiety disorder.

As a result, in children with fixed behavioral inhibition in different time periods, more anxiety disorder can be diagnosed, and more behavioral inhibition is observed in the children of individuals with anxiety disorder.

1.2.5. *Attachment*

In 1973, Bowlby [17] first mentioned the theory of attachment; in later years, Ainsworth [18] defined attachment to be categorized.

Accordingly, in the first year of life, a special relationship behavior develops between the baby and the primary caregiver. As a result of standardized behavioral observations (foreign status test), three types of attachment style are mentioned: (1), secure; (2), ınsecure avoidant; and (3), insecure disorganized.

Parents of children who are securely connected can have empathy with the needs of the child and are aware of their needs. The parents of unsafe children cannot do so.

Depending on the attachment style, the child learns cognitions about interpersonal relationships and develops strategies for emotion control. The child creates an internal working model. What is present in this model is the person he trusts and the world. The child thus evaluates situations and regulates interpersonal relationships. This study model, if it occurs, automatically processes and continues as fixed.

A secure attachment style is a protective factor in the development of anxiety. However, more actual studies should be conducted.

1.2.6. *Cognitive risk factors*

Cognitive perceptions play an important role in the development of anxiety disorders in children. In recent years, these cases have been specifically investigated. The extent to which the cognitive factors investigated is the risk factors.

1.2.6.1. *Control experiences in childhood*

Chorpita and Barlow [19] developed a model of vulnerabilities related to the emergence of fear and depression. According to this model, early uncontrollable and predetermined stimuli result in poor control experience and increased neurobiological activity and consequently behavioral inhibition system introduced by Gray. Neurobiological activation leads to indeterminate somatic symptoms that have been described for the first time by Kagan [9]. This diminishing control experience is a risk factor in difficult life events in the future. Physiological effects as well as weakened control experience lead to chronic cognitive deviations and result in fear-anxiety phenomenon. This uncontrollability and prior uncertainty are experienced in the early period with primary caregivers (e.g., weak empathy of parents) [8].

1.2.6.2. Anxiety sensitivity

According to the definition of anxiety sensitivity, anxiety and related symptoms (e.g., physical symptoms), while in a continuous state, cause physical, mental, or social problems [20]. Anxiety sensitivity is considered as a variable that emerges at different degrees compared to individuals. It can be affected by different factors. These factors may be genetic factors, life experiences, or panic attacks. The risk of recurrent panic attacks is increasing in new cases. Life experiences may lead to miscognitions (e.g., palpitation is a heart attack).

1.3. Summary and results

Anxiety disorders are early developmental, psychosocial, and psychopathological complications. Although early anxiety syndromes show spontaneous recovery, the majority of children and adolescents with anxiety disorders tend to experience new syndromes or other mental disorders in similar situations during their lifetime (other anxiety disorders, depressive disorders, or substance use). Secondary depressive disorders are a common complication. Detection of vulnerabilities and risk factors in the early period is also important in terms of development of programs aimed at conservation. Although some strong risk factors (parental attitudes, parental psychopathology, temperament alterations) have been identified, the recognition of the most powerful pectorists and the complex biological and psychological mechanisms should have implications for the development of anxiety disorder. Different risk factors play a role in different anxiety disorders. This situation also differs according to developmental periods.

Author details

Nese Kocabasoğlu[1] and R. Hülya Bingöl Çağlayan[2*]

*Address all correspondence to: rhulyabingol@gmail.com

1 Psychiatry Clinic, Istanbul University Cerrahpasa School of Medicine, Turkey

2 Children and Adolescent Psychiatry Clinic, Istnabul University Cerrahpaşa School of Medicine, Turkey

References

[1] Havighurst RJ. Research on the developmental-task concept. The School Review. 1956; **64**(5):215-223

[2] Waters E, Sroufe LA. Attachment as an organizational construct. In: Interpersonal Development. Routledge; 2017. pp. 109-124

[3] Gazelle H, Ladd GW. Anxious solitude and peer exclusion: A diathesis–stress model of internalizing trajectories in childhood. Child Development. 2003;**74**(1):257-278

[4] Walker EF, Diforio D. Schizophrenia: A neural diathesis-stress model. Psychological Review. 1997;**104**(4):667

[5] Kraemer HC, Kazdin AE, Offord DR, Kessler RC, Jensen PS, Kupfer DJ. Coming to terms with the terms of risk. Archives of General Psychiatry. 1997;**54**(4):337-343

[6] Last CG, Strauss CC. School refusal in anxiety-disordered children and adolescents. Journal of the American Academy of Child & Adolescent Psychiatry. 1990;**29**(1):31-35

[7] Last CG, Hersen M, Kazdin A, Orvaschel H, Perrin S. Anxiety disorders in children and their families. Archives of General Psychiatry. 1991;**48**(10):928-934

[8] Heim C, Nemeroff CB. The role of childhood trauma in the neurobiology of mood and anxiety disorders: Preclinical and clinical studies. Biological Psychiatry. 2001;**49**(12):1023-1039

[9] Kazdin AE, Kagan J. Models of dysfunction in developmental psychopathology. Clinical Psychology: Science and Practice. 1994;**1**(1):35-52

[10] Gest SD. Behavioral inhibition: Stability and associations with adaptation from childhood to early adulthood. Journal of Personality and Social Psychology. 1997;**72**(2):467

[11] Hirshfeld DR, Rosenbaum JF, Biederman J, et al. Stabile behavioral inhibition and its association with anxiety disorder. Journal of the American Academy of Child and Adolescent Psychiatry. 1992;**31**:103-111

[12] Matheny AP Jr. Children's behavioral inhibition over age and across situations: Genetic similarity for α trait during change. Journal of Personality. 1989;**57**(2):215-235

[13] Rosenbaum JF, Biederman J, Gersten M, Hirshfeld DR, Meminger SR, Herman JB, et al. Behavioral inhibition in children of parents with panic disorder and agoraphobia: A controlled study. Archives of General Psychiatry. 1988;**45**(5):463-470

[14] Rosenbaum JF, Biederman J, Hirshfeld-Becker DR, Kagan J, Snidman N, Friedman D, et al. A controlled study of behavioral inhibition in children of parents with panic disorder and depression. American Journal of Psychiatry. 2000;**157**(12):2002-2010

[15] Bowlby J. The making and breaking of affectional bonds: I. Aetiology and psychopathology in the light of attachment theory. The British Journal of Psychiatry. 1977;**130**(3):201-210

[16] Ainsworth MDS. The Bowlby-Ainsworth attachment theory. Behavioral and Brain Sciences. 1978;**1**(3):436-438

[17] Chorpita BF, Barlow DH. The development of anxiety: The role of control in the early environment. Psychological Bulletin. 1998;**124**(1):3

[18] Reiss S, Peterson RA, Gursky DM, McNally RJ. Anxiety sensitivity, anxiety frequency and the prediction of fearfulness. Behaviour Research and Therapy. 1986;**24**(1):1-8

[19] McNally RJ. Panic Disorder: A Critical Analysis. Guilford Press; 1994

[20] Reiss S. Theoretical issues in behavior therapy. Academic Press; 1985

[21] Noyes R, Crowe RR, Harris EL, Hamra BJ, McChesney CM, Chaudhry DR. Relationship between panic disorder and agoraphobia: A family study. Archives of General Psychiatry. 1986;**43**(3):227-232

[22] Fyer AJ, Mannuzza S, Chapman TF, Liebowitz MR, Klein DF. A direct interview family study of social phobia. Archives of General psychiatry. 1993;**50**(4):286-293

[23] Grillon C, Ameli R, Goddard A, Woods SW, Davis M. Baseline and fear-potentiated startle in panic disorder patients. Biological psychiatry. 1994;**35**(7):431-439

[24] Lewinsohn PM, Gotlib IH, Lewinsohn M, Seeley JR, Allen NB. Gender differences in anxiety disorders and anxiety symptoms in adolescents. Journal of abnormal psychology. 1998;**107**(1):109

[25] Federer M, Schneider S, Margraf J, Herrle J. Wie erleben achtjährige Panikanfälle? Wie erleben achtjährige Panikanfälle? 2000

[26] Hamm AO, Cuthbert BN, Globisch J, Vaitl D. Fear and the startle reflex: Blink modulation and autonomic response patterns in animal and mutilation fearful subjects. Psychophysiology. 1997;**34**(1):97-107

Section 2

The Epigenetics of Anxiety Disorders

Chapter 2

The Diaeventology of Anxiety Disorders

Daniel J. Guerra

Additional information is available at the end of the chapter

http://dx.doi.org/10.5772/intechopen.82176

Abstract

Anxiety is a crippling neuropsychiatric condition that encompasses a complex endophenotypic network of genetic, immunological, epigenetic, and metabolic mechanisms, interacting with the environment. A new approach to complex biological systems, including mental states and their neurological correlates, is diaeventology, a paradigm that exposes the event ontologies of these biomolecular/cellular mechanisms. General anxiety disorder has been studied in subclinical and clinical research settings where evidence is obtained for a longitudinal patterning of chronic and episodic and often increasingly stressful life events that provide the etiology and development of the pathology. Early events that involve brain oxygen deprivation coupled with carbon dioxide abundance are linked to biochemical and epigenetic processes associated with anxiety instantiation. A verified analysis of the current evidence suggests a neuroimmune mechanism that aligns with stress pathophysiology and epigenetic re-tailoring of key genomic loci that inappropriately compensate and misdirect biological defense mechanisms toward central nervous system dysfunction presenting as anxiety disorders.

Keywords: anxiety, diaeventology, genomics, epigenomics, neuroimmune

1. Introduction

Anxiety is associated with psychological states that consubstantially ignite an imbalance with the neuroimmune system. For example, cancer anxiety has been associated with a decrease in natural killer (NK) cells [1]. It is well established that care-givers of the terminally ill score higher than non-family members on the Hospital Anxiety and Depression Scale (HADS); but over time, this value decreases as the family member adapts to the worsening condition of their loved one [2]. These aspects of anxiety obtain neural correlates that are both endocrine stress hormone-linked and epigenetic in origin, with links to the immune system. Combined with an environment of stress, immune responses can epigenetically alter the expression of genetic loci and potentially modify those genes directly. This association of stress with later anxiety manifestation may have deeper roots going back to in utero events affecting the neuroimmunoepigenome of the fetus.

The interplay of organisms is the macrocosm, but it also appropriately describes the human body and overall stress imposed by the microbiome, invading pathogens, autoimmunity, cancer, autophagy, and senescence. The development, differentiation, and the signal transduction cascade network, including neuronal action potentials and endocrine mediation, also compose an opposing three-dimensional trigonal plane where the central element is the homeostasis of the existing individual. Indeed, learning and the accumulation of memories and knowledge are all part of a massive internal interactome that can be understood relative to advantage, vectorial control, and constant failure. Anxiogenesis can arise from perturbations to this system and manifest at the physiological and neuropsychological level.

There is a natural-native system that encompasses all of the features describing this neuropsychiatric interactome and its axis is the immune system. Thus, the immune system has two roles in the human body. One is for defense plus offense, and the other, in conjunction with epigenetic mechanisms, generates the existing individual. This is a perpetuating neural network that can learn, via attention and ascent to stress, to function within the world. Such a biologically adaptive phenomenon is accomplished via homologous recombination of variable regions of both the immunoglobulin family and the T-cell receptor in concert with chromatin remodeling, the histone code, and both the acetylome and methylome of cohering DNA. If there is a link between the mind and the body, at least one component is physical. This connection might be the molecular and cellular adaptive immunological interactome that serves to generate neural tracts according to developmental, endocrine, and peripheral stimuli while maintaining repair processes in the central nervous system (CNS) by using the complex interactions between microglia and neurons. Neural networks are processes, becoming eventual in nature, as contrasted with a substance ontology. The pattern of events appears as energetic fields rather than particles of matter, much like chemical bonds. An event ontology that reaches across the neural network of genetic and environmental interaction is articulated and synthesized through epigenetic modifications of the classical immune system, thus creating a responsive plastic and elastic memory field capable of learning, ideation, imagination, and understanding through time. This diaeventome involves the central existing individual agentically interacting through the events obtained across the inherited genome, the changing environment, and the transcendental immunoepigenome through time.

Figure 1 represents the current model.

This chapter will employ my new paradigm of diaeventology to introduce and instantiate the neural correlative endophenotype linked to the psychiatric condition general anxiety disorder (GAD).

Diaeventology (dialectical event ontology) is an adaptational, processive scientific accounting of the physiologico-rational human condition through cellular and molecular event ontology.

Its biological mechanism of action, linking pathopsychological states like GAD to biochemical pathways, incorporates the immuno-epigenomic induction of neural, endocrine, and

http://dx.doi.org/10.5772/intechopen.82176

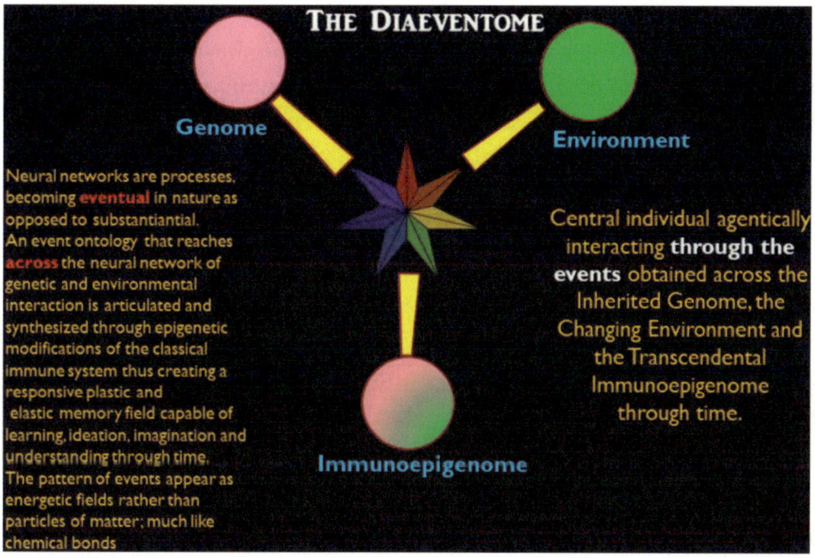

Figure 1. The diaeventome paradigm.

metabolic response to the micro- and macro-environment through classical constitutive-surveillance and acquired-effector cellular and humoral defense stratagems using reversible covalent modification and hydrophobic interactions of nucleic acids, proteins, and lipids.

Thus, I will explore how diaeventology offers a general molecular system theory for a free will-driven/agency-based individual adaptation and a knowledge-acquiring physiologico-rational mechanism that better explains the core event ontology of human existence including health and well-being.

2. Diaeventological sources of GAD

During early stages of embryo implantation, there is a suggested suppression of the immune response; yet, there are many immune systems at play. These include NK cells. NKs are innate immune cells that require no secondary or tertiary recombination and adaptation to kill target cells upon antigen presentation as with Major Histocompatibility Complex (MHC) class I-held antigens [3]. This allows NK cells to degranulate and release cytotoxic substances directly into targeted cells for destruction. There is a pull back, or switch, that may involve mesenchymal stem cells signaling through interferon that regulate and therefore license and delicense the NK killing based on chemokine reception and a global on/off switch [3].

A recent report catalogs some of the descriptors of immune surveillance in the uterus. In this chapter, it is reported that macrophages, NK cells, and T cells are found in the human decidua [3]. Over 70% of the detectable immune cells are NKs and the rest are mostly macrophages with small percentages of dendritic cells. They also summarize from the literature that no B or plasma cells can be detected. However, the remainder of the immune cell population is of T-cell lineage.

Of interest to the argument that the diaeventome drives an epigenetically modifiable immune-based regulation of global physiological and pathophysiological consequence is that the ablation of NK cells prevents trophoblasts from obtaining endometrial vascularity. This results in spontaneous abortion. Whether this phenomenon is associated with controlled cell destruction or chemokine/cytokine-mediated signaling, leading to reprogramming of gene expression, is not yet clear, but it does suggest that NK cells may be necessary for in utero trophoblast invasion. Since dendritic cells play a key role in communication between the constitutive and adaptive immune response, it is of further note that loss of uterine Dendritic Cell (DCs) blocks decidual maturation and blastocyst implantation [3].

Stress can induce epigenetic changes to loci that control the expression of RNAi production. RNAi epigenetics involves the production of interfering RNA species and thus prevents target mRNA expression. This removal of target mRNA can have global or specific effects on gene expression including those involved in psychiatric and mood disorders [4].

Even though chronic psychological and social stress has been implicated in anxiety disorders, the mechanism for how social defeat and worrying can be linked to genomic or epigenomic phenomena has been difficult to track.

Recently, it was reported that chronic stress in a murine model was targeting an RNASE II enzyme complex (DROSHA subunit) via differential hypomethylation at that locus. A decrease in methylation suggests there is a concomitant increase in the non-specific expression of the target gene, and in this case, it would mean an increase in RNAi-mediated epigenetic ablation of gene expression [5].

In a rat model, pro-inflammatory CNS-localized M1 type microglia are induced by cumulative unpredictable mild stress (CUMS) within the Hypothalamic Pituitary Adrenal (HPA) axis [6]. This resulted in the expression of pro-inflammatory tumor necrosis factor (TNF)-α, interferon (INF)-γ, interleukin (IL)-1β, and IL-17 cytokines while simultaneously reducing the production of the anti-inflammatory IL-4, IL-10, and IL-13 cytokines typically associated with the regulatory M2 microglial lineage [6].

Macrophages are classified into inflammatory or anti-inflammatory. Inflammatory macrophages differentiate in response to microbial and tumor antigens and interferon γ by producing pro-inflammatory cytokines at the site of nascent infection and cancerous lesions while anti-inflammatory macrophages differentiate via signaling by glucocorticoids or anti-inflammatory (type II) cytokines like IL-4, IL-13, and IL-10 where they promote TH2 immunity and mediate tissue remodeling, wound healing, and immune modulation [7].

The cytokines IL-4 and IL-13 drive anti-inflammatory macrophage polarization through the IL-4 receptor alpha chain (IL-4Rα), and anti-inflammatory polarization is also promoted by activation of several master regulators, including signal transducer and activator of transcription 6 (STAT6), Krüppel-like factor 4 (KLF4), and interferon regulatory factor 4 (IRF4) [7].

Diet and nutritional life style choices likely modulate macrophage polarization and, by inference, the inflammatory response associated with anxiety disorder. Bioenergetic reprogramming is associated with this mechanism wherein the inflammatory macrophage cell type is fueled by aerobic glycolysis and can be triggered by the bacterial antigen LPS ± the pro-inflammatory cytokine IFN-γ. Within the anti-inflammatory lineage, IL-4 induces the expression of PPARγ which in turn transcriptionally activates the urea cycle enzyme arginase 1 (Arg1) and the β-oxidation of fatty acids along with electron transport chain/oxidative phosphorylation gene expression and an increased capacity for mitochondrial biogenesis [7]. To fuel the anti-inflammatory bioenergetics, IL-4 also induces expression of CD36 which acts as a membrane receptor for circulating LDL and very low density lipoprotein (VLDL)-rich triacylglycerol (TAG). Finally, the unloading of triacylglycerol (TAG) and associated fatty acid hydrolase activity is linked to fatty acid oxidation, thus completing the anti-inflammatory polarization phenotype [7].

Recently, a macrophage-specific cytokine has been linked to anxiety. The macrophage migration inhibitory factor (MIF) is a pro-inflammatory macrophage-specific cytokine that is active in the HPA axis and characterized haplotype variants of that gene were linked to diminished expression and lowered adolescent anxiety disorder [8]. MIF has been linked to the recruitment of natural killer T cells via an IFN-γ gradient in skin lesions, thus suggesting a similar role in causing the migration and stimulation of inflammatory leucocytes in the HPA axis [9]. Indeed, MIF has been implicated with this dual cytokine/chemokine role in a large cluster of inflammatory diseases, thus suggesting a global immunopathological association of macrophages and other leucocytes in neuropsychiatric disease [10]. A previous report suggested that deletion or pharmacological inhibition of MIF biological activity in the hippocampal gyrus of mice resulted in anxiety-like behavior and this was correlated with a lack of neurogenesis in the region [11].

Combined, this evidence on macrophage switching, inflammation, and neurogenesis (thus targeting the canonical HPA axis) all point to a diaeventological progression of both environmental and genetic plus epigenetic event ontologies that instantiate a temporal link to anxiety disorders.

3. Acquired neuroimmune responses and GAD

The serotonin transporter (HTTPLPR) has been linked to depression and GAD in human populations. The short allele of the HTTPLPR gene was associated with these neuropsychiatric disorders although whether there was a hypo- or hyper-HPA axis effect depended upon the cohort population under study including parameters age, race, and gender [12]. However, this is not necessarily ambiguous, since the downstream processing of serotonin binding to its receptor is complicated by the level of allele-specific HTTPLPR-mediated translocation, availability of serotonin, plus the receptor subtype, and ultimate release of glucocorticoid via the HPA axis [12].

There are serotonin receptors on macrophages, monocytes, and lymphocytes, and these subpopulations interact to mediate inflammatory responses leading to HPA axis activity [13].

Serotonin has been associated with a blockade of the antigenic determinate capacity of macrophages via IFN-γ, thus diminishing the suppression of NK cells and therefore enhancing their potential cytotoxic function on host cells [13].

For their part, NK cells contribute to inflammation via their frank cytotoxicity, thus releasing potential activating antigens of pathogenic origin. NK cells also establish and maintain the "cytokine storm" which lays out the persistence and maturation of the local inflammatory response [14]. Certain non-cytotoxic clones of NK cells over-express high IFN-γ while others, that are manifestly cytotoxic, produce negligible amounts of IFN-γ. A third sub-population of NKs weighs in with intermediate characteristics [14].

Upon signaling-based activation, NKs kill their target via direct cellular contact involving either secretory lysosomal cytotoxic perforin and granzymes or deployment of the "death receptors and ligands" such as FasL and TRAIL, which mediate target cell apoptosis [14]. This shift to NK cell plenary function can mediate effects in the HPA that could result in either attenuation or enhancement of glucocorticoid signaling that would impact GAD and Major Depressive Disorder (MDD).

While these interacting immune responses maintain a metastable inter-uterine environment, the successful development of the fetus requires a perpetual modification of the mechanism that must deliver a balance between surveillance of potential toxic stress metabolites and pathogens on one hand, and the tolerance of the developing baby on the other.

Consequently, the presence of immune cells at the implantation site is not associated with a response to the "foreign" fetus but to facilitate and protect the pregnancy. Therefore, it should be theorized that the immune system at the implantation site is not suppressed; on the contrary, it is active and functional and is carefully controlled via real-time procession of gene expression—controlled by the developmental program between mother and fetus and the epigenetic modifications that are necessary for signal response (including stress) from the entire biological system including the external environment.

4. Epigenetics of the early uterine environment and potential for GAD imprinting

Anxiety disorder is clearly associated with biochemical and cellular phenomena. The interactions between the genome and the environment are well described and paradigmatic in the biomedical literature. However, the link to behavioral and neuropsychiatric disorders has been more recent and the inclusion of the epigenome is particularly compelling.

Genetic and "epigenetic" mechanisms shape biological activity and can respond negatively to produce the pathophysiological state. While the mammalian genome establishes the template for empirically discernable developmental and behavioral patterns, a more complex and variable phenomenon helps to produce the final phenotype. This latter "epigenetic" mechanism has increasingly become the subject of developmental and cell biology, gene expression, and disease. The biochemistry of epigenetics involves several covalent modifications of nuclear chromatin as well as post-transcriptional gene silencing [15].

Among these modifications is the methylation of the C5 atom on cytosine residues found in certain canonical CpG islands associated with promoter elements. Methylation, acetylation, ubiquination, and phosphorylation of cohering histones and the processing of double-stranded RNA in the generation of siRNA are epigenetic phenomena involved in the modulation of gene expression. The mechanisms of these epigenetic phenomena have been described and they include the activities of methyltransferases, acetyltransferases, kinases, phosphatases, demethylases, deacetylases, E3 ubiquitin ligases, and RNase enzymes [16]. The substrates for these reactions are either chromatin or in the case of the RNase activities, double-stranded mRNA. S-adenosyl methionine (SAM or AdoMET) is the recognized nuclear methylation agent, deriving the methyl group from folic acid derivatives. Acetyl CoA is used in acetylation of chromatin-associated histones in the process of chromatin remodeling which generally enhances gene expression downstream from ligand/receptor-mediated activation of the complex which may be in association with the nuclear ubiquitin/proteasomal pathways. Nuclear-associated posttranslational modifications (such as acetylation) of histone carboxyl termini clearly alter chromatin structure and function [16]. The major effect is a pronounced change in the physical-chemical accessibility of DNA-binding proteins to unwind the double helix and potentiate the transcription to RNA. These covalent modifications are at least conceptually reversible, but often, they can lead to a complete removal of histones from the chromatin complex, thus inducing for a time in the cell cycle, uncontrolled constitutive gene expression. Indeed, while methylation tends to dissociate histones from the chromatin complex, demethylation tends to favor non-transcribable chromatin rearrangement although this leaves open the potential for acetylation which often promotes chromatin remodeling and gene expression [16].

Besides the specificity of the methyltransferases and acetyl transferases on certain histone residues (typically LYS), there is also a specificity at the amino acid sequence level. To generate changes in reactivity of chromatin to remodeling, only certain covalently modified histone amino acid residues play a role. The discrete biochemistry of these epigenetic modifications are lysine methylation, acetylation and ubiquination, serine phosphorylation, and arginine methylation. All of these modifications have been observed by superimposition of the diet (see below). The point is that, these covalent modifications effect DNA accessibility to various proteins and they alter protein:protein interactions among chromatin-bound histones and other polypeptides [16].

The "histone code" hypothesis asserts that covalent modification of chromatin-bound histones is communicated to a host of nuclear proteins to provide a directive for discrete chromatin molecular dynamics and gene expression control. The theory suggests that other proteins and protein complexes can distinguish and indeed interpret histone modifications. Communication of the histone code to the nuclear machinery of transcription ultimately controls gene expression or silencing, heterochromatin formation, DNA replication, and even chromosome segregation [16]. All of these mechanisms play a diaeventological role in neuropsychiatric states such as anxiety.

Most if not all of these epigenetic modifications are heritable changes in gene expression. Even though DNA sequence modification does not generally occur, there are reports where amplification of nucleotide repeats can be proximal to DNA methylation. Whether or not this is a common phenomenon in acquired epigenesis may be significant in neuropsychiatric disease. What is clear is that many developmental disorders as well as cancer, age-related illnesses, and various brain disorders are linked to changes in DNA methylation. Epigenetic modifications (especially DNA methylation) provide a fine tuning on gene expression. Induced hypermethylation by xenobiotics as well as hypomethylation are linked to these diseases [16].

Besides involvement in various diseases, epigenetic phenomena are developmentally programmed. As such, epigenetic control over gene expression and cell differentiation as well as tissue formation and neurogenesis has been extensively reported. Epigenetics also plays a major role in immune response. In fact, mechanisms including CpG methylation and various histone modifications are basic biochemical phenomena regulating the mammalian immune response. Chromatin remodeling as well as the cohering epigenetic control over transcriptional processes have been shown to help regulate cytokine expression and secretion as well as antigen processing and T-cell differentiation. In this way, environmentally controlled epigenetic mechanisms as well as the methylation state of the immune cell chromatin are involved in the differentiation of T helper cells which in turn activate both T-cell and B-cell-mediated acquired immunity [17].

Since it is well documented that epigenetics plays a role in emotions and behavior, the link between immune response and emotions such as anger, depression, and anxiety has both a strong theoretical and empirical basis. I have previously discussed the role of cytokines in inducing the RAGE circuitry [15]. As it turns out, transcriptional control over cytokine gene expression is a key element in the regulation of the immune response. One of the transcription factor proteins that play a role in this regulation includes nuclear factor-kappaB (NF-kappaB) which is necessary for the innate immune response as well as T-cell differentiation, which is the cellular basis of acquired immunity. Environmental control over NF-kappaB transcriptional, post-transcriptional (mRNA processing and siRNA), and post-translational modifications is integral to both immune systems. This global control over cytokine expression and release as conferred by the NF-kappaB transcription factor has been termed the "enhanceosome." Epigenetic phenomena including stress play a large role in the immune-associated control over cellular differentiation including that occurring in the mammalian brain [18].

Covalent epigenetic modifications have a profound influence over gene expression and the mechanism for this effect requires environmental input and readily available substrates including target DNA and associated histones plus the methylating agent. During fetal development, it has been shown that obese pregnant mothers can pass on a pro-obese phenotype to their offspring. It has been known for some time that maternal metabolism during gestation has an imprinting effect on fetal gene expression. Indeed, this epigenetic regulation controls the divergent expression of paternal over maternal genes including one involved in glucose metabolism and growth, the insulin-like-growth factor 2 (IGF2) [19]. This fetal imprinting is the result of maternal metabolism which is indirectly linked to maternal diet. This epigenetic effect is presumed advantageous during a specific stage of gestation. However, if these epigenetic modifications sustain into later stages of gestation, they may run the risk of being a component of "maintenance methylation" which persists after parturition and into infancy, childhood, and even adult development. This may predispose the individual to new environmental pressures leading to chronic diseases such as obesity, metabolic syndrome, and cardiovascular and renal dysfunction. There is no reason to avoid speculation on these mechanisms and other disease states such as GAD.

Besides the gestational effects of maternal obesity on subsequent metabolic dysfunction in the offspring, nutritional deficiencies or excesses can also specifically alter the epigenome. Dietary sources of methylating agents such as bioavailable folic acid, methionine, choline, betaine, and homocysteine may have a permanent effect on the epigenetic methylation patterns of CpG islands and cohering histones in locus and temporal-dependent genes [20]. If these gene products are involved in normal development and have been arbitrarily altered, the fetus may not develop correctly or there may be infant diseases linked to these methylation patterns. As the individual matures to adulthood, the maternal exposure to methyl-group-containing nutrients may have a life-long effect on basic physiology, response to nutrition, and, sometimes, pathological and disease states [20].

The mechanism of chromatin methylation involves a group of enzymes. Some function directly on cytosine residues in double-stranded chromatin DNA. These DNA methyltransferases (DNMT1, DNMT3a, and DNMT3b) establish specific signatures or patterns and one of the isoforms, DNMT1, maintains the methylation and preferentially recognizes hemi-methylated DNA as substrate, thereby establishing second strand complementary methylation and a germline transference of the pattern after DNA replication [20]. It has been demonstrated that hyperinsulinemia coupled with hyperglycemia, two common outcomes in metabolic syndrome will increase the activity of DNMT and cause a general increase in hepatic DNA methylation [21]. This enhancement of DNA methylation is a direct consequence of increased flux through the homocysteine ➔ methionine ➔ adoMet pathway via an increase in both homocysteine methylation and the adoMet synthase [16].

As mentioned above, the predisposition to chronic diseases such as obesity and metabolic syndrome may arise in utero via the fetal programming mechanism. A study that examined intrauterine growth retardation in rats showed that a homeobox gene (Pdx1) became hypermethylated and therefore silenced and this led to offspring with diabetes type II disease [22]. Pdx1 is a transcriptional regulator gene involved in pancreatic beta cell functioning. In utero methylation of this gene was linked to the activity of histone deacetylase activity (HDAC 1), suggesting cross-talk in the epigenomic programming. Indeed, an increase in HDAC1 activity caused deacetylation of key histones that subsequently became methylated along with the proximal promoter region of Pdx1. This methylation pattern was conferred to the offspring and Pdx1 was completely silenced in these diabetes type II rats, suggesting that control over both DNA methylation and histone code in utero could be the direct cause of beta cell dysfunction leading to hyperinsulinaemia in the offspring [22]. It should be noted that growth retardation, as used in this study, would limit the level of growth hormone (GH) to the developing fetus. Growth hormone is secreted by the pituitary upon stimulation by the starvation hormone acyl ghrelin. Hyperinsulinaemia and gestational diabetes have been linked to childhood anxiety.

In a recent report, glucose metabolism as controlled by PDX-1-linked insulin sensitivity was linked to anxiety in an animal model [23]. This diaeventomic combination of genomic X environmental X neuroimmunoepigenomic modulation provides the molecular mechanism linking numerous childhood diseases with stress, pain, and anxiety including a strong correlate to basic human needs such as nutrition and pain avoidance.

Clearly, diet plays a major role in both general and specific epigenomic patterns and these can cause significant metabolic diseases.

Diet, both at the caloric and nutrient levels, controls metabolic flux in a dynamic way. Excess caloric intake can induce several disease states including obesity and the metabolic syndrome. Insufficient caloric intake can also cause disease as can inappropriate nutrition or excessive digestion of vitamins and certain growth-promoting molecules. Besides a direct effect on metabolic rate and function, diet can also introduce these epigenetic changes to the endocrine hormone system.

Genetic mutations that are acquired somatically can be passed on to subsequent generations and these are most commonly in the form of single nucleotide polymorphisms (SNPs) or in some, perhaps, rarer instances, copy number variations (CNVs). Once these genetic mutations have occurred and DNA has gone through a round of replication, they remain more or less fixed in the genome and become correlated with anxiety [24].

The most common cause of these genetic mutations is some kind of physical or chemical damage to the DNA as can be acquired by inflammation or environmental toxins including radiation from the sun in the form of unprotected UV light.

The epigenetic mutations on the other hand can arise within a single generation and remain fixed there, or in the mechanism of maintenance methylation, they can also be preserved and inherited. Therefore, the distinction between the two forms of modification lies more in the degree of alteration in gene expression than in the mechanisms of acquisition or potential for inheritance. Indeed, environment plays a very significant role in epigenesis of the endocrine system and may be the more robust factor in variations around this physiological axis [16]. Since the endocrine hormones play such a major role in anxiety disorders, the connection to methylation is robust.

As mentioned above, the degree of DNA or histone methylation is somewhat dependent upon the availability of biological methylating agents at the site of reaction. Therefore, adoMET and folic acid levels can be linked to the titration of these covalent modifications. The key to understand epigenetic changes is the degree of such events during critical periods of development and in particular during disease states that impact metabolism through endocrine control. Another key feature of epigenetic changes vs. genetic is the reversibility of the former and the stability of the latter. Epigenetic changes that include DNA methylation, histone acetylation, methylation, and the expression of small interfering RNA have the largest impact on protein levels and can therefore exert more profound control over metabolism than genetic modifications which may or may not effect protein expression or function [16].

It is conceivable that the mammalian uterus has an active licensing program that is involved in selective killing of certain cell masses, for example, the decidua. This would allow for preferential embryo adherence and implantation so that the initial phases of the mammalian gestation can proceed. As it turns out, sirtuin-mediated control over the interferon pathway may coordinate this licensing. The literature on this subject directs toward creating viral-free zones all the way through placental genesis that is mediated by this epigenetic reprograming (licensing) of NK cells [25]. But, maybe this is not for antiviral purposes. In fact, interferon can be stimulated by cytosolic chromatin DNA in the form of mini-chromosomes that are the result of chromatin interrogation during times of epigenetic reprogramming [26]. This (now) cytosolic DNA triggers the interferon gamma pathway which in turn is precipitated and processed by nuclear exposure of endogenous retrovirus expression and DNA accumulation into satellite DNA endosomes via sirtuin-mediated changes in acetylation [26].

The tolerance of the fetus occurs during human gestation and could be linked to in utero epigenetic mechanisms that ultimately result in the potential for GAD in the adolescent or adult. Clearly, a diaeventomic mechanism is at play in the neuroimmunoepigenome, and imprinting of neuropsychological traits might have origins in utero.

This epigenetic reformation and realignment of the developmental program as directed by stress requires not only differential changes in multiple gene axes within cell masses embedded in complex tissues and organs including circulating leucocytes but also the bioenergetic requirements of such cells to mediate proliferation and exposure to noxious environments [27, 28].

It has been established that the switch from carbohydrate to fatty acid as the major biofuel is linked with central and peripheral inflammation. Both glycolysis and fatty acid beta-oxidation work in tandem to provide reducing equivalents for the electron transport chain and the proton pumping mitochondrial ATPase [27, 28].

Such early life adversities (ELFs) as maternal stress during pregnancy have been correlated to both anxiety disorders and the potential for the experience of pain throughout life. A recent paper has linked animal model carbon dioxide exposure and subsequent hypersensitivity to ELF-associated anxiety [29]. In this study, mice were cross-fostered in an atmosphere enriched to 6% CO_2 in the presence or absence of an acid channel ion sensing 1 gene (ACIS1) blockade drug called amiloride. When the drug was nebulized vs. administered via injection, a decrease in anxiety disorder behavior was observed. Previous work had shown an epigenetic modification of the ACIS1 expression via CO_2 enrichment that was correlated with animal distress. Indeed super-elevated concentrations of atmospheric CO_2 tend to generate a powerful pain and anxiety state in model animals and in human subjects. The link to ACIS1 expression alteration due to epigenetic modification of mRNA levels, in response to elevated CO_2, suggests this increase in gene expression is a protective response. This is a combined chemoreceptive/nociceptive stress-induced molecular modification that has been observed in the medulla oblongata where the protection centers around the response to CO_2-induced cerebral acidosis that leads to ACIS1-protective modification in respiration and nociception. Where epigenetically predisposed GAD and panic disorders are correlated with elevated CO_2 levels as induced in utero or as the result of ELF-associated choking or suffocation, the blockade of the ACIS1 gene with amiloride may be considered as a potential pharmacotherapeutic intervention [29]. The key point derived from this study is that environmental stress induces a neuroepigenomic response that may instantiate pCO_2 levels and reconditioning toward psychiatric conditions (e.g., GAD) in adults. In a study involving over 170 college-aged subjects that were genotyped according to 11 potential endogenous biomarker polymorphisms, the respiratory hypersensitivity to elevated CO_2

levels was statistically correlated to the ASIC1 common gene variant (rs1108923). This heritable variant thus segregated with a general anxiety and panic disorder-linked respiratory endophenotype [30]. Whether this gene variant would be either sufficient or necessary for respiratory distress-linked anxiety was not addressed. Upon consideration of the pathophysiological response and potential for genetic and epigenetic diaeventological interactions, it is at best a correlation that requires careful experimentation before validation of the argument.

Traumatic brain injury (TBI) is a tremendous health issue worldwide and is responsible for a considerable amount of brain-associated permanent disability and death. While physical blunt force trauma is a major source of TBI, CO_2 intoxication is also a contributing factor. Hyperbaric partial pressure of CO_2 in the blood (paCO2) alters the autoregulation of blood flow to the brain [31]. Blood vessels in the CNS respond to O_2, CO_2 and pH, and mediate mean arterial pressure (MAP) within a short window (50–150 mmHg). When MAP falls above or below this range, the capacity for autoregulation collapses and either hypotensive ischemia or hypertensive edema can result [31].

These conditions can occur in utero and throughout the post gestational life. This effectively induces neuroimmune activation that can be modified via epigenetic mechanisms leading in some instances to a potential for predisposition to GAD and other neuropsychiatric disorders. Clearly a case for a diaeventological mediated pathophysiological state.

In the specific case of $paCO_2$ effects on autoregulation, decreases cause vasoconstriction while an increase in this parameter is associated with vasodilation of the cerebral blood vessels [31]. This response is acutely sensitive to $paCO_2$ because CO_2 dissolves far better than O_2 in aqueous. However, the $paCO_2$ effect is directed to control the paO_2 for cerebral oxygen demand which is essential to prevent brain damage and death. O_2 consumption in the brain is linked to neuronal and microglial activity. As neuronal action potentials fire, this increases biological demand for O_2 to drive ATP production via metabolism and the electron transport chain/ oxidative phosphorylation (ETC/OXPHOS) [31]. Both catecholamines and excitatory amino acids will increase O_2 demand and if blood flow is restricted due to the $paCO_2$, the relative concentration of neurotransmitters increases, thus potentiating neuronal damage and microglial activation to generate pro-inflammatory cytokines. When $paCO_2$ is increased, another problem arises, and this involves the increase in intracranial pressure because of excessive blood flow. This is similar to stroke associated with edema that results in the extravasation of vessel contents into surrounding tissues, thus causing an increase in interstitial fluid which will induce an immune response [31].

Increases or decreases in CO_2 levels in the brain can result in neuroimmune activation that can lead to HPA axis stimulation and ultimately the endophenotypes linked to anxiety disorders. When this occurs chronically during gestation, the fetus may obtain epigenetic alterations in key metabolic, hormonal, and immune pathways leading to a predisposition to anxiety disorders in adulthood. Likewise, this can be repeated during early infant and childhood development, and into adulthood.

5. The diaeventological axis

Living systems interact according to a three-dimensional biological trigonal plane according to the square of opposition:

A. Universal affirmative: No harm to host(s); maximum benefit to both; rare or occasional dependence.

E. Universal negation: Severe harm to hosts; benefit to only 1 host; 100% dependence.

I. Particular affirmative: benefit is disinterested; 50% dependence.

O. Particular negation: Some harm to neither; benefit to neither; no dependence for either.

This interplay involves the macrocosm, but it also appropriately describes the microcosm (human body and overall stress) imposed by the microbiome, invading pathogens, autoimmunity, cancer, autophagy, and senescence. This is the mechanism by which neuropathology is established in the CNS as described for example in glioblastoma [32].

Development, differentiation, and the signal transduction cascade network, including neuronal action potentials, neuroimmune mechanisms, and endocrine mediation, compose an opposing three-dimensional trigonal plane where the central element is the homeostasis of the existing individual.

Indeed, learning and the accumulation of memories and knowledge are all part of a massive internal interactome that can be understood compared to advantage, vectorial control, and constant failure and compensation. This is the basis for diaeventology as introduced in the introduction of this chapter.

There is a natural-native system that encompasses all of these features: the immune system.

Thus, the immune system has two roles in the human body. One is for defense and the other, in conjunction with epigenetic mechanisms, generates the existing individual with an ongoing neural network that can learn, via attention and ascent to stress on the system. This is accomplished via homologous recombination of variable regions of both the immunoglobulin family and the T-cell receptor in concert with chromatin remodeling [33], the histone code, and both the acetylome and methylome of cohering DNA [34].

If there is a link between the double aspect of mind and the body, at least one component is physical. This connection might be the molecular and cellular adaptive immunological interactome that serves to generate neural tracts according to developmental, endocrine, and peripheral stimuli, while maintaining repair processes in the CNS, by using the complex interactions between microglia and neurons.

It is well established that neuroinflammatory mediators play a critical role in the pathophysiology of brain ischemia, exerting either deleterious effects on the progression of tissue damage or beneficial roles during recovery and repair [35].

The immune response could function to generate the networked synaptic connections in the brain during development and throughout life. Soon after an ischemic insult, increased levels of cytokines and chemokines enhance the expression of adhesion molecules on cerebral endothelial cells. This causes the adhesion and transendothelial migration of circulating neutrophils and monocytes [36]. These immune cells may accumulate in the capillaries, decreasing cerebral blood flow. They can further extravasate into the brain parenchyma, thus impacting neuropsychiatric states [37].

Besides this, the infiltrating leukocytes, as well as resident brain cells, (neurons and macrophage-like microglia) may release pro-inflammatory agents like cytokines, chemokines, and oxygen/nitrogen radicals that result in tissue damage [38]. Moreover, recent studies have highlighted the involvement of matrix metalloproteinases in the propagation and regulation of neuroinflammatory responses to ischemic brain injury. These enzymes cleave protein components of the extracellular matrix such as collagen, proteoglycan, and laminin, but also process a number of cell-surface and soluble proteins, including receptors and cytokines such as interleukin-1β, thus promoting CNS inflammation and the potential for anxiety disorders [39].

The innate immune cells, macrophages, are classified into inflammatory or anti-inflammatory. Inflammatory macrophages differentiate in response to microbial and tumor antigens and interferon γ by producing pro-inflammatory cytokines at the site of nascent infection and cancerous lesions [40].

Anti-inflammatory macrophages differentiate via signaling by glucocorticoids or anti-inflammatory (type II) cytokines like IL-4, IL-13, and IL-10 where they promote TH2 immunity and mediate tissue remodeling, wound healing, and immune modulation.IL-4 and IL-13 drive anti-inflammatory macrophage polarization through the IL-4 receptor alpha chain (IL-4Rα), and anti-inflammatory polarization is also promoted by activation of several master regulators, including signal transducer and activator of transcription 6 (STAT6), Krüppel-like factor 4 (KLF4), and interferon regulatory factor 4 (IRF4), thus implicating all of these proteins in control over the generation of anxiety [40].

Macrophage polarity and activation are linked to neuropsychiatric conditions including GAD and MDD. A case in point is acute respiratory distress syndrome (ARDS) [41].

Acute respiratory distress syndrome (ARDS) is associated with an imbalance in the level of respiratory oxygen intake and CO_2 release and thus is linked to known potential pathophysiological states and GAD. ARDS can be fatal if not treated appropriately. In adults, it is associated with stiffness of the respiratory system evident in the pulmonary oxygenation step. This results in both chronic and acute hypoxemia. ARDS pathology is characterized by injury to the capillary endothelia and subsequent damage to alveoli, severe arterial vasoconstriction, and pulmonary hypertension [42]. Subsequent to lung injury, ARDS patients are typically treated with granulocyte/macrophage colony stimulating factor (GM-CSF) as a component of their pharmacotherapy [41].

GM-CSF is a pro-inflammatory cytokine associated with enhancing the level of circulating leucocytes while decreasing fetal hemoglobin levels in sickle cell anemia patients, making it a potential target for blockade with pharmacological agents [43].GM-CSF is linked to decreased oxygenation in the blood and increased immune activity-associated inflammation. While GM-CSF was also linked to depression and anxiety score elevation in ARDS patients, corticosteroids, which reduce the inflammatory response, had the opposite effect on these disorders [41].GM-CSF expression is stimulated by pro-inflammatory cytokines and inhibited by anti-inflammatory cytokines and also serves to both stimulate and regulate pro-inflammatory cytokines, thus suggesting a direct role in the activation of type I macrophages, which have been linked to GAD and associated depressive disorders [44].

Bioenergetic reprogramming is associated with macrophage polarization. The inflammatory macrophage cell type is fueled by aerobic glycolysis and can be triggered by LPS ± IFN-γ. With the anti-inflammatory lineage, IL-4 induces the expression of PPARγ, which in turn transcriptionally activates the urea cycle enzyme arginase 1 (Arg1), and the β-oxidation of fatty acids (Beta-OX) along with ETC/OXPHOS increased capacity via mitochondrial biogenesis. To fuel the anti-inflammatory bioenergetics, IL-4 also induces expression of CD36 which acts as a membrane receptor for circulating low-density lipoprotein (LDL) and VLDL-rich TAG. Finally, the unloading of TAG and associated fatty acid hydrolase activity is linked to Beta-OX, thus completing the anti-inflammatory polarization [40]. Inhibiting neuroinflammation has become a new strategy in biological psychiatry.

A recent report examines the use of a potential probiotic bacterium, *Mycobacterium vaccae* NCTC 11659 [45]. *M. vaccae* could become a biological means to treat anxiety disorders and its mechanism may involve the enhancement of T regulatory cells (T_{reg}) which act to curtail T-effector (T_{eff}) cell-meditated inflammation via the stimulation of anti-inflammatory cytokines such as IL-10, and TGF-β regionally in the hippocampus. Whether biofuel switching plays a role in this response has not been fully addressed, but elsewhere it has been reported that T_{reg}-cell metabolism toward Beta-OX and lipid utilization enhances the T_{reg} control over T_{eff}-cell-mediated inflammatory responses and further that T_{eff} cells tend to use aerobic glycolysis over Beta-OX [46].

Besides neuronal firing, hormonal signaling, cell transduction cascades, cytokine and chemokine synthesis and release, and immune cell epigenetic patterning, this biofuel connection to anxiety disorders helps to explain how in utero dietary fluctuations can affect the developing fetus.

6. Conclusions

The pre-programming of the neuroimmuno epigenome may be one of the pillars of longitudinal psychiatric disease development. A diaeventological paradigm is thus developing to explain the biological patterning of anxiety disorders. **Figure 2** below provides a developmental time course for the molecular and cellular GAD patterning described in the text.

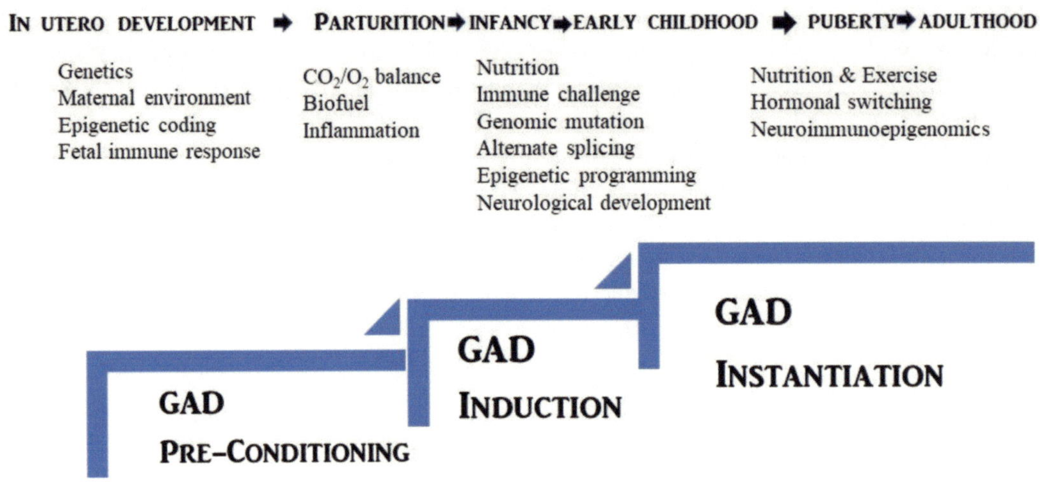

Figure 2. The diaeventomic development of anxiety disorders.

Acknowledgements

The author wishes to acknowledge his family for their support.

Conflict of interest

The author claims no conflict of Interest.

Author details

Daniel J. Guerra

Address all correspondence to: djgphd@gmail.com

VerEvMed LLC, Juliaetta, Idaho, USA

References

[1] Koga C, Itoh K, Aoki M, Suefuji Y, Yoshida M, Asosina S, et al. Anxiety and pain suppress the natural killer cell activity in oral surgery outpatients. Oral Surgery, Oral Medicine, Oral Pathology, Oral Radiology, and Endodontics. 2001;**91**(6):654-658. DOI: 10.1067/moe.2001.115465

[2] Lee Y, Lin P-Y, Chien C-Y, Fang F-M, Wang L-J. A comparison of psychological well-being and quality of life between spouse and non-spouse caregivers in patients with

head and neck cancer: A 6-month follow-up study. Neuropsychiatric Disease and Treatment. 2018;**14**:1697-1704. DOI: 10.2147/NDT.S162116

[3] Mor G, Cardenas I. The immune system in pregnancy: A unique complexity. American Journal of Reproductive Immunology. 2010;**63**(6):425-433. DOI: 10.1111/j.1600-0897.2010.00836.x

[4] Miller BH, Wahlestedt C. MicroRNA dysregulation in psychiatric disease. Brain Research. 2010;**1338**:89-99. DOI: 10.1016/j.brainres.2010.03.035

[5] Kocak EE. RNA interference: A new hope in understanding and treatment of psychiatric disorders. Bulletin of Clinical Psychopharmacology. 2012;**22**(4):366-374. DOI: 10.5455/bcp.20120731055453

[6] Zhang C, Zhang Y-P, Li Y-Y, Liu B-P, Wang H-Y, Li K-W, et al. Minocycline ameliorates depressive behaviors and neuro-immune dysfunction induced by chronic unpredictable mild stress in the rat. Behavioural Brain Research. Jan 1 2019;**356**:348-357 DOI: 10.1016/j.bbr.2018.07.001

[7] Kang S, Nakanishi Y, Kioi Y, et al. Semaphorin 6D reverse signaling controls macrophage lipid metabolism and anti-inflammatory polarization. Nature Immunology. 2018;**19**(6):561-570. DOI: 10.1038/s41590-018-0108-0

[8] Lipschutz R, Bick J, Nguyen V, Lee M, Leng L, Grigorenko E, et al. Macrophage migration inhibitory factor (MIF) gene is associated with adolescents' cortisol reactivity and anxiety. Psychoneuroendocrinology. 2018;**95**:170-178. DOI: 10.1016/j.psyneuen.2018.05.033

[9] Hsieh CY, Chen CL, Lin YS, Yeh TM, Tsai TT, Hong MY, et al. Macrophage migration inhibitory factor triggers chemotaxis of CD74+CXCR2+ NKT cells in chemically induced IFN-γ-mediated skin inflammation. Journal of Immunology. 2014;**193**(7):3693-3703. DOI: 10.4049/jimmunol.1400692

[10] Klasen C, Ohl K, Sternkopf M, et al. MIF promotes B cell chemotaxis through the receptors CXCR4 and CD74 and ZAP-70 signaling. Journal of Immunology. 2014;**192**(11):5273-5284. DOI: 10.4049/jimmunol.1302209

[11] Conboy L, Varea E, Castro JE, Sakouhi-Ouertatani H, Calandra T, Lashuel HA, et al. Macrophage migration inhibitory factor is critically involved in basal and fluoxetine-stimulated adult hippocampal cell proliferation and in anxiety, depression, and memory-related behaviors. Molecular Psychiatry. 2011;**16**(5):533-547. DOI: 10.1038/mp.2010.15

[12] Carbia C, López-Caneda E, Corral M, Cadaveira F. A systematic review of neuropsychological studies involving young binge drinkers. Neuroscience and Biobehavioral Reviews. 2018;**92**:338-349. DOI: 10.1016/j.neubiorev.2018.04.013

[13] Herr N, Bode C, Duerschmied D. The effects of serotonin in immune cells. Frontiers in Cardiovascular Medicine. 2017;**4**(48). DOI: 10.3389/fcvm.2017.00048

[14] Cribbs A, Hookway ES, Wells G, et al. Inhibition of histone H3K27 demethylases selectively modulates inflammatory phenotypes of natural killer cells. The Journal of Biological Chemistry. 2018;**293**(7):2422-2437. DOI: 10.1074/jbc.RA117.000698

[15] Guerra DJ, Colonnello V, Panksepp J. The neurobiology of RAGE and anger & psychiatric implications with a focus on depression. In: Pahlavan F, editor. Psychology of Emotions, Motivations and Actions. Multiple Facets of Anger: Getting Mad or Restoring Justice? Hauppauge, NY: Nova Science Publishers; 2011. pp. 45-79

[16] Carbonell A, Fueyo R, Izquierdo-Bouldstridge A, Moreta C, Jordan A. Epigenetic mechanisms in health and disease: BCEC 2017. Epigenetics. 2018;**13**(3):331-341. DOI: 10.1080/15592294.2018.1434391

[17] Sawalha AH. Epigenetics and T-cell immunity. Autoimmunity. 2008;**41**(4):245-252. DOI: 10.1080/08916930802024145

[18] Vanden Berghe W, Ndlovu MN, Hoya-Arias R, Dijsselbloem N, Gerlo S, Haegeman G. Keeping up NF-kappa B appearances: Epigenetic control of immunity or inflammation-triggered epigenetics. Biochemical Pharmacology. 2006;**72**(9):1114-1131. DOI: 10.1016/j.bcp.2006.07.012

[19] Godfrey KM, Reynolds RM, Prescott SL, et al. Influence of maternal obesity on the long-term health of offspring. The Lancet Diabetes & Endocrinology. 2017;**5**(1):53-64. DOI: 10.1016/S2213-8587(16)30107-3

[20] Zeisel SH. Epigenetic mechanisms for nutrition determinants of later health outcomes. The American Journal of Clinical Nutrition. 2009;**89**(5):1488S-1493S. DOI: 10.3945/ajcn.2009.27113B

[21] En-Pei IC, Yi-Cheng W, Wei-Wen C, Feng-Yao T. Effects of insulin and glucose on cellular metabolic fluxes in homocysteine transsulfuration, remethylation, S-adenosylmethionine synthesis, and global deoxyribonucleic acid methylation. The Journal of Clinical Endocrinology and Metabolism. 2009;**94**(3):1017-1025. DOI: 10.1210/jc.2008-2038

[22] Park JH, Stoffers DA, Nicholls RD, Simmons RA. Development of type 2 diabetes following intrauterine growth retardation in rats is associated with progressive epigenetic silencing of Pdx1. The Journal of Clinical Investigation. 2008;**118**(6):2316-2324. DOI: 10.1172/JCI33655

[23] Yu J, Liu SH, Sanchez R, Nemunaitis J, Brunicardi FC. Hypoglycemia and PDX1 targeted therapy. Journal of Endocrine Disorders. 2015;**2**(1):1018

[24] Guerra D. The neurobiology of anger involving medical, pharmacological and neuroimmune implications. Chapter 5. In: Cruz JFA, Sofia RMC, editors. Anger and Anxiety: Predictors, Coping Strategies, and Health Effects. Nova Publishers; 2017. ISBN: 978-1-53612-932-8

[25] He Y, Tian Z. NK cell education via nonclassical MHC and non-MHC ligands. Cellular & Molecular Immunology. Hauppauge, NY. 2017;**14**:321-330. DOI: 10.1038/cmi.2016.26

[26] Dou Z, Ghosh K, Vizioli MG, et al. Cytoplasmic chromatin triggers inflammation in senescence and cancer. Nature. 2017;**550**(7676):402-406. DOI: 10.1038/nature24050

[27] Feldman EL, Bennett DLH, Nave K-A, Jensen TS. New horizons in diabetic neuropathy: Mechanisms, bioenergetics, and pain. Neuron. 2017;**93**(6):1296-1313. DOI: 10.1016/j.neuron.2017.02.005

[28] Xu WD, Yang XY, Li DH, et al. Up-regulation of fatty acid oxidation in the ligament as a contributing factor of ankylosing spondylitis: A comparative proteomic study. Journal of Proteomics. 2015;**113**:57-72. DOI: 10.1016/j.jprot.2014.09.014

[29] Battaglia M, Rossignol O, Bachand K, D'Amato FR, De Koninck Y. Amiloride modulation of carbon dioxide hypersensitivity and thermal nociceptive hypersensitivity induced by interference with early maternal environment. Journal of Psychopharmacology (Oxford, England). 2018 Jun 1:269881118784872. DOI: 10.1177/0269881118784872

[30] Savage JE, McMichael O, Gorlin EI, et al. Validation of candidate anxiety disorder genes using a carbon dioxide challenge task. Biological Psychology. 2015;**109**:61-66. DOI: 10.1016/j.biopsycho.2015.04.006

[31] Battisti-Charbonney A, Fisher J, Duffin J. The cerebrovascular response to carbon dioxide in humans. The Journal of Physiology. 2011;**589**(Pt 12):3039-3048. DOI: 10.1113/jphysiol.2011.206052

[32] Pawlowska E, Szczepanska J, Szatkowska M, Blasiak J. An interplay between senescence, apoptosis and autophagy in glioblastoma multiforme—role in pathogenesis and therapeutic perspective. International Journal of Molecular Sciences. 2018;**19**(3):889. DOI: 10.3390/ijms19030889

[33] Bassing CH, Swat W, Alt FW. The mechanism and regulation of chromosomal V(D)J recombination. Cell. 2002;**109**((2) Supplement 1):S45-S55. DOI: 10.1016/S0092-8674(02)00675-X

[34] Janssen KA, Sidoli S, Garcia BA. Recent achievements in characterizing the histone code and approaches to integrating epigenomics and systems biology. Methods in Enzymology. 2017;**586**:359-378. DOI: 10.1016/bs.mie.2016.10.021

[35] Shichita T, Sakaguchi R, Suzuki M, Yoshimura A. Post-ischemic inflammation in the brain. Frontiers in Immunology. 2012;**3**:132. DOI: 10.3389/fimmu.2012.00132

[36] Kim ND, Luster AD. The role of tissue resident cells in neutrophil recruitment. Trends in Immunology. 2015;**36**(9):547-555. DOI: 10.1016/j.it.2015.07.007

[37] de Oliveira S, Rosowski EE, Huttenlocher A. Neutrophil migration in infection and wound repair: Going forward in reverse. Nature Reviews Immunology. 2016;**16**(6):378-391. DOI: 10.1038/nri.2016.49

[38] Wang WY, Tan MS, Yu JT, Tan L. Role of pro-inflammatory cytokines released from microglia in Alzheimer's disease. Annals of Translational Medicine. 2015;**3**(10):136. DOI: 10.3978/j.issn.2305-5839.2015.03.49

[39] Rempe RG, Hartz AM, Bauer B. Matrix metalloproteinases in the brain and blood-brain barrier: Versatile breakers and makers. Journal of Cerebral Blood Flow and Metabolism. 2016;**36**(9):1481-1507. DOI: 10.1177/0271678X16655551

[40] Kang S, Nakanishi Y, Kioi Y, et al. Semaphorin 6D reverse signaling controls macrophage lipid metabolism and anti-inflammatory polarization. Nature Immunology. 2018;**19**(6):561-570. DOI: 10.1038/s41590-018-0108-0

[41] Spencer-Segal JL, Hyzy RC, Iwashyna TJ, Standiford TJ. Psychiatric symptoms in survivors of acute respiratory distress syndrome. Effects of age, sex, and immune modulation. Annals of the American Thoracic Society. 2017;**14**(6):960-967. DOI: 10.1513/AnnalsATS.201606-468OC

[42] Umbrello M, Formenti P, Bolgiaghi L, Chiumello D. Current concepts of ARDS: A narrative review. International Journal of Molecular Sciences. 2017;**18**(1):64. DOI: 10.3390/ijms18010064

[43] Ikuta T, Adekile AD, Gutsaeva DR, et al. The proinflammatory cytokine GM-CSF downregulates fetal hemoglobin expression by attenuating the cAMP-dependent pathway in sickle cell disease. Blood Cells, Molecules & Diseases. 2011;**47**(4):235-242. DOI: 10.1016/j.bcmd.2011.08.005

[44] Bhattacharya P, Budnick I, Singh M, et al. Dual role of GM-CSF as a pro-inflammatory and a regulatory cytokine: Implications for immune therapy. Journal of Interferon & Cytokine Research. 2015;**35**(8):585-599. DOI: 10.1089/jir.2014.0149

[45] Reber SO, Siebler PH, Donner NC, et al. Immunization with a heat-killed preparation of the environmental bacterium mycobacterium vaccae promotes stress resilience in mice. Proceedings of the National Academy of Sciences of the United States of America. 2016;**113**(22):E3130-E3139. DOI: 10.1073/pnas.1600324113

[46] Galgani M, De Rosa V, La Cava A, Matarese G. Role of metabolism in the immunobiology of regulatory T cells. Journal of Immunology. 2016;**197**(7):2567-2575. DOI: 10.4049/jimmunol.1600242

Section 3

Different Types of Anxiety Disorders

Chapter 3

Dental Anxiety and Its Consequences to Oral Health Care Attendance and Delivery

Irene Kida Minja and
Febronia Kokulengya Kahabuka

Additional information is available at the end of the chapter

http://dx.doi.org/10.5772/intechopen.82175

Abstract

Dental anxiety has been reported to be a common problem affecting widespread societies, hence a global public health concern. This chapter provides an updated information to dental practitioners, about dental anxiety and its implication to oral health-care attendance and service delivery. It is introduced by defining dental anxiety, providing a summary of prevalence of the problem among children and adults; and its relationship with sociodemography, oral health status, and cultural issues. Causes of dental anxiety and simple ways to diagnose it and management options of dental anxiety for different age groups of populations are summarized to assist dental practitioners during patient management. How dental anxiety influences dental attendance and ultimately impact oral health status of populations; and its relationship with oral health-care delivery are also discussed. Finally, preventive measures both in community and clinical settings are provided and recommendation for dental professionals and other stake holders is outlined.

Keywords: dental anxiety, oral health-care delivery, oral health-care attendance

1. Introduction

1.1. Definition

The terms dental anxiety, fear, and phobia, though often used mutually, differ depending on the situation within which they occur. Nevertheless, a distinction has been made between these terminologies. *Dental fear* is a reaction to a known danger, which involves a "fight-or-flight" response when confronted with a threatening stimulus. On the other hand, *dental anxiety* is a reaction to an unknown danger, and *dental phobia* is basically the same as fear, only much stronger, whereby the "fight-or-flight" response occurs when just thinking about or being reminded of the threatening situation [1].

Dental anxiety is extremely common, and most people experience some degree of the anxiety especially if they are about to have a certain dental procedure done which they have never experienced before. Moreover, someone with a dental phobia will avoid dental care at all costs until either a physical problem or the psychological burden of the phobia becomes overwhelming. In this chapter, the term dental anxiety is employed.

1.2. Prevalence of dental anxiety

Dental anxiety is reported to be a global public health concern due to its effects on individual's oral health and quality of life. The prevalence of the condition in children ranges from 5 to 61% [2, 3] and in adults from 1 to 52% [4–12], inclusive of participants with both moderate and high dental anxiety.

1.3. Factors associated with dental anxiety

1.3.1. Sociodemographics

A majority of studies done reveal that females of all age groups, younger age and people who are classified to have low level of education are at more risk of having dental anxiety [2, 11]. The main reasons cited for the observed differences are more linked to environmental factors rather than biological makeup among children. However, Folayan and coworkers [13] revealed no differences in the prevalence of dental anxiety with sociodemography in children, while Minja et al. [11] showed no sex difference in their study among adults.

1.3.2. Oral health status

Individuals with poor oral health status are reported to perceive dental anxiety than their counter parts with good oral health status. Clinically, these patients are observed to have high number of decayed and missing teeth and less restored teeth [14–16]. DeDonno [17] revealed an association between participants' dental anxiety and oral hygiene, whereby individuals with dental anxiety were seen to have poor oral hygiene. Furthermore, patients who are dentally anxious are usually least satisfied with the appearance of their teeth [18].

1.3.3. Oral health-related behaviors

Population studies show that individuals with dental anxiety have difficulties to attend to a dentist [19]. Dental anxiety has also been reported to impact on individuals' daily living including modification of eating habits, such as avoidance of hard to chew and foods that cause sensitivity. Further to this, individuals with dental anxiety are reported to have a high tendency to self-medication so as to avoid visiting a dentist [20].

1.3.4. Cultural issues

The role of culture and norms in modifying individual's perception of dental fear and anxiety is also of prime importance when explaining these phenomena. Culture has been reported to have influence on perceiving dental anxiety [21]. Studies have shown that dental anxiety expression significantly varied according to ethnicity as well as religion due to the engraved dental anxiety coping mechanisms and expression among different cultures [22]. Generally, it has been reported that societies with cultures that emphasize on greater self-control, emotional restraint, and compliance to social rule (such as some Asian and African countries) were more likely to score higher in their fears/anxiety [23].

2. What is dental anxiety

In order to understand the dental anxiety well, it is important to explain its pathway, causes, diagnosis, and management.

2.1. Dental anxiety pathway

Five theories are thought to better explain the pathways of dental anxiety: *Pavlovian cognitive conditioning, informative pathway, vicarious conditioning, verbal transmission/threat, and parental pathway* [24].

Pavlovian cognitive conditioning is the most commonly utilized pathway of dental fear and anxiety used by the patients, whereby past painful dental experience may negatively impact an individuals' future dental attendance.

Informative pathway is an indirect pathway to phobia that involves learning about fearful dental events as told by other individuals.

Vicarious conditioning is another indirect pathway, whereby individuals may acquire dental phobia by learning indirectly through observing the responses of others attending a dentist.

In *Verbal transmission/threat*, there is no direct observation of traumatic/fearful event, but through hearing or reading about dangerous or threatening information about a stimulus irrespective of an actual presence of the threating stimulus. In this pathway, dental visit is used as a disciplinary measure for misbehaving.

Parental pathway refers to a situation where a fearful behavior displayed by a parent becomes a pathway of acquiring dental anxiety by a child. A stronger relationship is observed when it is the mother who expresses intensified fearful behavior.

2.2. Causes of dental anxiety

Dental anxiety has a wide range of causes and hence it is considered complex and multifactorial [25]. The causes may be patient, provider, or environment related. The patient-related causes include past dental experience, pain, influence of family, or peer experience and personality, whereas provider-related causes include communication techniques and provider's bad behavior. Environmental-related causes include sounds of drills or other apprehensive patients, unpleasant smell/clinic area, and sight of blood or local anesthetic injections [26].

2.3. Diagnosis of dental anxiety

The importance of proper diagnosis of dental anxiety cannot be underrated. Identifying anxious patients helps a dental care provider to plan for appropriate ways and procedures for managing the patient. Several means have been developed to identify patients who have dental anxiety before treatment is initiated, so as to assist a dentist to provide appropriate treatment with no negative consequences to both the patient and provider. The measures are grouped into two: *use of questionnaires* and *objective measures* of dental anxiety.

2.3.1. Use of questionnaire

Using reliable and easy-to-administer tools for assessment of dental anxiety at the dental setting is beneficial for the dental team [27]. Despite the presence of a number of pretreatment questionnaires for patient administration, very few dental health-care providers utilize them [28]. Using self-reported questionnaire has been reported to be useful to assist in disclosing as well as reducing dental anxiety, as it might be a way for the dental team to gently build rapport with a patient [29]. A number of self-rated tools are available and no single instrument can be regarded as a gold standard set of questions. Mentioned here are the most commonly used and have shown acceptable psychometric properties for use in different languages worldwide. These measures are simple, easy to use, and acceptable to both patients and dental team [30–32]. They include a four-item Corah's dental anxiety scale (CDAS) and a five-item modified dental anxiety scale (MDAS) which proved to be suitable for use among adults. The results can be utilized in grouping patients according to the level of dental anxiety that is *low, moderate,* and *high*. Other measures suitable for use among children are the modified child dental anxiety scale (MCDAS) containing eight questions; and a faces version of the modified child dental anxiety scale (MCDASf) that incorporates facial images on the response format, and this can be used by children as young as 3 years old [27, 29]. Use of questionnaires assists in identifying patients with dental anxiety thus allows planning for possible approaches that can be utilized for management of patients, as suggested by Newton and coworkers [33].

2.3.2. Objective measures

Measuring patients' vital signs can add into the identification of patients with dental anxiety at the dental clinic setting. These measures are assessment of blood pressure, pulse rate, pulse oximetry to assess blood oxygen levels which is affected by stress and anxiety, finger temperature, and galvanic skin response that measures skin conductance of weak electric current [29, 34].

2.4. Management of dental anxiety

When managing a patient with dental anxiety, utilization of different measures to counter anxiety will depend on the patient's history, age, and cooperation. In all instances, a dental care provider needs to portray behavior that will contribute to reducing anxiety to the patient. These include, but not limited to, being composed and relaxed, friendly to the patient, avoiding being judgmental or instilling pain, being supportive and encouraging to the patient, and working efficiently [26, 29]. Different measures are employed in managing patients with dental anxiety as explained below according to the age group of the patient.

2.4.1. Management in children

In managing children with dental anxiety, the following is suggested:

- Allocate enough time for appointment.
- Communicate effectively.
- Utilize the four "s" principle by reducing triggers of stress. These are *sight* of injections, handpieces, and blood; *smell* of materials such as eugenol; *sound* of drilling or other patients crying; and *sensation* of vibrating instruments.
- Distract the patient using music, video.
- Give a sense of control over the procedure by involving the patient during treatment, like to raise hand when feeling pain or uncomfortable.
- Reduce pain by giving enough anesthesia.
- Provision of cognitive behavioral therapy (CBT).
- Provision of relaxation therapy for older children that will assist patients to gain control over their psychological state. The techniques can be given before and even during the procedure. These may include *Jacobsen's progressive muscular relaxation, paced breathing techniques*.

In highly anxious patients who could not do any of the psychotherapeutics, pharmacotherapy may be indicated such as:

- Conscious sedation technique, whereby drugs are provided to render an anxious patient to a depressive state. The routes of application can be oral, sublingual, intramuscular, rectal, and in dental setting with enough resources, intravenous administration, or inhalation using nitrous oxide (N_2O) gas.
- When the above techniques do not help, the practitioner can refer the patient to a specialist psychologist for further management or can resort to general anesthesia if equipment and trained personnel are available.

2.4.2. Management in adults and older adults

All the techniques used in children can be utilized when managing adults with dental anxiety. In addition, the following techniques can be employed:

- Utilization of computer-assisted relaxation learning (CARL), which is a self-paced treatment by patients to cope with dental anxiety (needle specific) without the presence of a therapist.

- Individual systematic desensitization, whereby patients are gradually introduced to a fearful stimulus and learn to cope with anxiety by utilizing another method such as CARL or relaxation therapy methods.
- For patients whose anxiety is induced by a needle, computer-controlled local anesthesia can be used; or electronic dental anesthesia, wherein anesthesia is achieved based on "gate-control theory of pain," with no use of a needle. This method, though, is expensive and requires special training.
- Adults could also be referred for group therapy with specialist psychologist and behavioral therapist.

2.4.3. Benefits to patients

A patient will calm down, hence be receptive of oral health information provided for his/her own benefit. Furthermore, the patient will allow receiving the required treatment. Ultimately, the patient will be positively motivated, on a long-term basis and thus acquire positive attitudes toward dentistry.

2.4.4. Benefits to practitioner

This will assist service provider to be at peace, hence facilitate accurate provision of the required treatment. The whole scenario will, eventually, minimize occupational stress.

3. Dental anxiety and its consequences to oral health-care attendance and delivery

Generally, dental procedures take a couple of minutes to accomplish, and therefore require a patient to be calm and cooperative in the dental chair. Unfortunately, this is not always the case, since some patients are apprehensive probably because most procedures are either believed or are actually associated with some degree of pain to the patient. Furthermore, dental patients are usually "alert" or "not ill," thus in full perception of all that is happening. This situation contributes to acquisition of dental anxiety.

3.1. Influence of dental anxiety on dental attendance and oral health status

It has been observed that individuals with dental anxiety tend to fail to keep appointments, avoid attending to a dentist for dental care or complying with prescribed treatment [35]. This tendency cuts across all individuals regardless of their socioeconomic status or geographical location. Dental anxiety is also associated with poor dental health conditions [36]. Research shows that anxious patients possess poor oral health when compared to nonanxious counterparts in terms of decayed, missing, and filled teeth [37]. Moreover, poor oral health conditions negatively impact individuals' quality of life [38, 39]. Generally, dental anxious patients have been viewed as unreliable and of poor economic risk [26].

The cycle of dental anxiety (**Figure 1**) explains the interrelationship of the above. Whereby, an individual with dental anxiety is usually worried and anticipates that something bad is going to happen if she/he visits a dentist; thenceforth, tends to delay or avoid dental attendance. This action deprives the individual from receiving dental preventive care and treatment and thus leads to deterioration of oral health, poor oral health status, and poor dental-related quality of life. Poor oral health, coupled with feeling of guilt, shame, inferiority, and worry of being reprimanded by a dentist for oral neglect, further increases dental anxiety and the cycle continues [40, 41]. Failure to provide the required treatment to counter dental anxiety, the vicious cycle will continue. It has been suggested that effective treatment of dental anxiety will improve dental attendance and ultimately the oral health of individuals [42].

3.2. Influences of dental anxiety on oral health-care delivery

Good oral health-care delivery entails harmonious environment contributed to by both providers and patients as well as dental environment. When either party's attributes are not positive toward reaching a harmonious environment, it may interfere with attaining the intended management goals.

3.2.1. Provider perspective

Provider's good communication skills coupled with proper use of behavior management techniques as well as positive behavior toward dental patients play a significant role in creating a harmonious dental treatment environment. The reverse may induce dental anxiety or exacerbate the already anxious situation [43]. Ultimately, treatment may take longer or may have to be rescheduled but may also be compromised. Various consequences of this situation include loosing patients, bad provider reputation, and negative professional image, as well as negative economic implications. Consequences affecting the patient directly include eliciting pain and

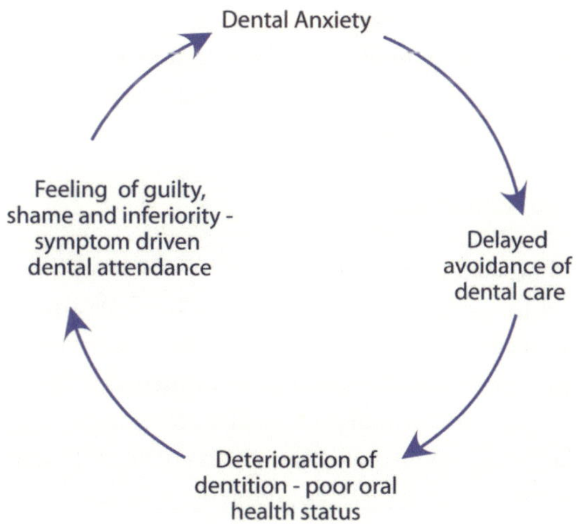

Figure 1. The vicious cycle of dental anxiety [40, 41].

contributing to patients' unpleasant dental experience. Handling an anxious patient when not prepared has been reported to add stress on the dentist and the dental team as a whole [44].

3.2.2. *Patient perspective*

Delaying, rescheduling, or avoiding dental visit due to dental anxiety leads to seeing a dentist only when it is inevitable, which may end up into a need for complicated treatment [36]. The latter might bring about more anxiety, failure to abide to instructions, or comply to preventive care hence exaggerate oral health problems [43]. Unfortunately, causes of dental anxiety such as personality, past dental experience, or family/peer influence are basically out of patients' control. Therefore, they need to be assisted to overcome the anxiety, which is a sole responsibility of the dental team. The dental team should have a broad approach on patient's needs, not be judgmental while managing the patient, instead do all that is required to allay the patient's anxiety, thus facilitating provision of proper care.

3.2.3. *Environmental perspective*

Dental environment is generally perceived by patients to be unfriendly, offensive, and anxiety-provoking, especially so by anxious patients. The looks of the dental chair and its accessories may not give an appealing first impression. Smell of the medicaments as well as invasive contact in the mouth, sound of the drill, sight of blood are some of the situations that most patients may have difficulties to tolerate [45]. The dental environment condition, coupled with the nature and duration of dental treatment procedures, may bring about or amplify patient dental anxiety. This situation will interfere with delivery of dental care. It is, therefore, the responsibility of the dental team to make sure that the dental environment is friendly to patients with or without dental anxiety.

3.3. Prevention of dental anxiety

Like in any other disease/condition, prevention before development of dental anxiety is important for effective management of patients. This may entail putting in place modifications to address operators, patients, or dental clinic environment concerns. Further to this, strategies aiming at the community may be critical.

3.3.1. *Modification of operator characters*

Operators/dental team character plays a big role in determining future behavior of dental patients. Particularly, what the patient experiences at his/her first visit to a dentist is what shapes his/her attitudes with dental care services [46]. Positive behavior of operator and the dental team will automatically influence positive attitudes and minimize chances for dental anxiety. On the contrary, a bad operator/dental team behavior may induce, as well as exaggerate, dental anxiety in patients [43, 47]. To prevent operators/dental team from inducing dental anxiety, starting from the moment the patient enters the dental clinic to exiting, it is advisable for the team to have good communication skills, be sympathetic, have empathy, and be able to control temper. To make this happen, proper training and continuing education on prevention of dental anxiety are of paramount importance. Therefore, the provider and dental team at large should strive to intentionally acquire these characteristics, which will lead to having positive behavior toward patients, particularly to be understanding to anxious ones.

3.3.2. Modification of patient characters

Every dental patient has his/her own preconceived ideas about dental care. Apparently, each patient might be anxious depending on his/her personality trait, past dental experience, influence from family and peers, etc. Therefore, all patients attending the dental clinic should be calmed down and be made to relax regardless of whether the patient is anxious or not, (**Figure 2a** and **b**). This is a sole responsibility of the dental team [48].

3.3.3. Modification of dental clinic environment

Most patients consider the dental environment to be unfriendly and anxiety provoking. For this reason, various efforts have been made by dental professionals to modify the environment so as to counter that effect (**Figures 3** and **4**). The efforts include avoiding white uniforms by using attractive colorful attire, minimizing bright lights, playing soft/relaxing music, placement of nondental attractions in waiting rooms, making reception and waiting rooms colorful for children, minimizing noise from dental instruments/equipment by sound proofing the operating rooms, and intentionally engaging a receptionist who is charming, positive, and having caring attitudes to patients. Other measures are utilization of aromatherapy and sensory-adapted dental environment (SDE). Aromatherapy in dental settings is done using essential oils, the most common ones being smell of orange and lavender. Lavender smell has been shown to produce positive physiological and pharmacological effects which proved to

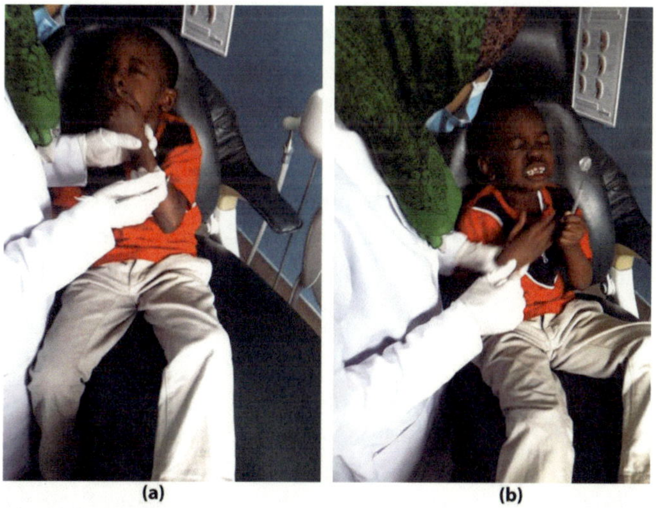

Figure 2. (a) A 7-year-old child presenting with dental anxiety trying to stop the doctor from performing oral examination. (b) The same child while a dentist employs behavior management techniques to allay the child's dental anxiety (pictures by courtesy of Dr. Gustav Rwekaza).

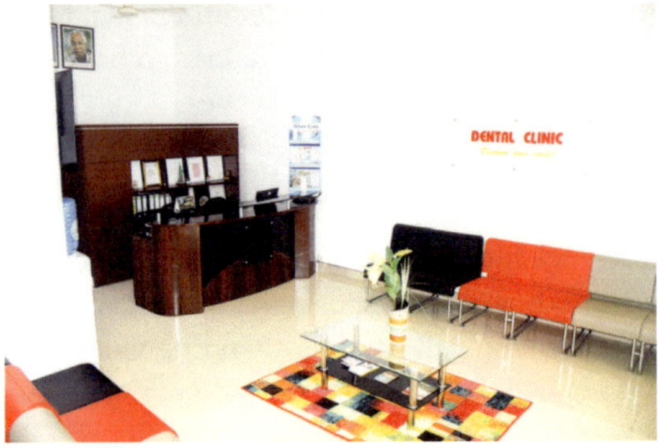

Figure 3. A patient-friendly dental clinic reception (picture by Jacob Francis, courtesy of Smiles dental clinic).

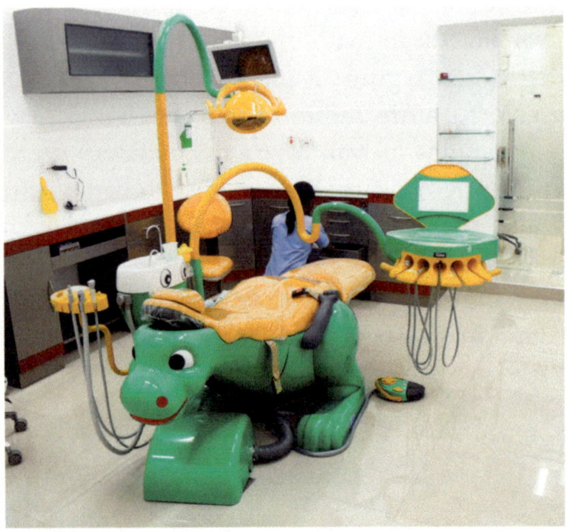

Figure 4. A child-friendly dental surgery (picture by Jacob Francis, courtesy of Smiles dental clinic).

be effective in reducing state anxiety [49]. Similarly, SDE, which has been utilized and proved to be effective for management of dental anxiety, is also helpful in reducing the anxiety and relaxing the patient [45].

3.3.4. Community prevention

At community level, prevention of dental anxiety through giving education is a responsibility of the dental team. The education should primarily be directed to children since the onset of dental anxiety often occurs in childhood. This implies that early intervention will help to prevent the problem from extending into adulthood, but adults should also be involved. Among measures of intervention at community level, it is to inform the community on the impact of dental anxiety on individual's oral health status, oral health-care attendance, and service delivery. Another measure is to educate and discourage individuals from sharing their dental fears and/or negative dental experiences in such a way that it may influence others to develop

http://dx.doi.org/10.5772/intechopen.82175

dental anxiety or negativity toward dentistry. Furthermore, it is beneficial to empower the community to prevent dental diseases, to encourage them on the importance of regular visit to a dentist for checkup, and to strongly disapprove the use of dental visit/services as punitive measure or to shape behavior [24, 48]. Moreover, population screening for dental anxiety will assist in identifying those who are affected thus earmarking them for preventive intervention.

4. Conclusions

Dental anxiety is a problem affecting populations of all ages, from all geographical locations. It affects individuals' oral health status, interferes with dental attendance and service delivery. Dental professionals, therefore, have a major role to play in the management and prevention of dental anxiety among dental patients and the community at large.

5. Recommendations

We recommend that:

1. Dental professional associations and dental teaching institutions should conduct workshops and continuing education and professional development (CPD) courses for the dental fraternity on management and prevention of dental anxiety.
2. Dental professionals to educate themselves on the different options of management and prevention of dental anxiety.
3. Dental professionals to educate community on dental anxiety.

Acknowledgements

Authors acknowledge funding support by Swedish International Development Agency (Sida) through Muhimbili University of Health and Allied Sciences (MUHAS).

Conflict of interest

The authors of this chapter declare no conflict of interest.

Author details

Irene Kida Minja* and Febronia Kokulengya Kahabuka

*Address all correspondence to: ikminja@gmail.com

Muhimbili University of Health and Allied Sciences (MUHAS), Dar es Salaam, Tanzania

References

[1] Armfield JM. Towards a better understanding of dental anxiety and fear: Cognitions vs. experiences. European Journal of Oral Sciences. 2010;**118**(3):259-264

[2] Klingberg G, Brogerg A. Dental fear/anxiety and dental behaviour management problems in children and adolescents: A review of prevalence and concomitant psychological factors. International Journal of Paediatric Dentistry. 2007;**17**(6):391-406. DOI: 10.1111/j.1365-263X.2007.00872.x

[3] Bhola R, Malhotra R. Dental procedures, oral practices, and associated anxiety: A study on late-teenagers. Osong Public Health and Research Perspectives. 2014;**5**(4):219-232. Available from: https://www.sciencedirect.com/science/article/pii/S2210909914000654

[4] Coolidge T, Hillstead MB, Farjo N, Weinstein P, Coldwell SE. Additional psychometric data for the Spanish modified dental anxiety scale, and psychometric data for a Spanish version of the revised dental beliefs survey. BMC Oral Health. 2010;**10**:12

[5] Akarslan Z, Erten H, Uzun O, Iseri E, Topuz O. Relationship between trait anxiety, dental anxiety and DMFT indexes of Turkish patients attending a dental school clinic. Eastern Mediterranean Health Journal. 2010;**16**(5):558-562. Available from: http://apps.who.int/iris/handle/10665/117916

[6] Humphris G, King K. The prevalence of dental anxiety across previous distressing experiences. Journal of Anxiety Disorders. 2011;**25**(2):232-236

[7] Arigbede A, Ajayi D, Adeyemi B, Kolude B. Dental anxiety among patients visiting a university dental centre. Nigerian Dental Journal. 2011;**19**:20-24. Nigerian Dental Association

[8] Coker A, Sorunke M, Onigbinde O, Awotie A, Ogubanjo O, Ogubanjo V. The prevalence of dental anxiety and validation of the modified dental anxiety scale in a sample of Nigerian population. Nigerian Medical Practitioner. 2012;**62**:5-6. Available from: https://www.ajol.info/index.php/nmp/article/view/93818

[9] Koleoso O, Akhigbe K. Prevalence of dental anxiety and the psychometric properties of modified dental anxiety scale in Nigeria. World Journal of Dentistry. 2014;**5**(1):53-59

[10] Appukuttan D, Subramanian S, Tadepalli A, Damodaran LK. Dental anxiety among adults: An epidemiological study in South India. North American Journal of Medical Sciences. 2015;**7**(1):13-18

[11] Minja IK, Jovin AC, Mandari GJ. Prevalence and factors associated with dental anxiety among primary school teachers in Ngara district, Tanzania. Tanzania Journal of Health Research. 2016;**18**(1):1-10

[12] Mehta N, Arora V. Prevalence of dental anxiety among patients visiting the out patient department (OPD) of a dental institution in Panchkula, Haryana. International Journal of Health Sciences and Research. 2017;**1**(7):27-33. Available from: http://www.ihrjournal.com/index.php/ihrj/article/view/57

[13] Folayan M, Idehen E, Ufomata D. The effect of sociodemographic factors on dental anxiety in children seen in a suburban Nigerians hospital. The Journal of Clinical Pediatric Dentistry. 2003;**13**(1):20-26

[14] Kruger E, Thomson W, Poulton R, Davies S, Brown R, Silva P. Dental caries and changes in dental anxiety in late adolescence. Community Dentistry and Oral Epidemiology. 1998; **26**(5):355-359. DOI: 10.1111/j.1600-0528.1998.tb01973.x

[15] Schuller AA, Willumsen T, Holst D. Are there differences in oral health and oral health behavior between individuals with high and low dental fear? Community Dentistry and Oral Epidemiology. 2003;**31**(2):116-121. DOI: 10.1034/j.1600-0528.2003.00026.x

[16] Eitner S, Wichmann M, Paulsen A, Holst S. Dental anxiety—An epidemiological study on its clinical correlation and effects on oral health. Journal of Oral Rehabilitation. 2006;**33**(8): 588-593. DOI: 10.1111/j.1365-2842.2005.01589.x

[17] Ma DD. Dental anxiety, dental visits and oral hygiene practices. Oral Health & Preventive Dentistry. 2012;**10**(2):129-133. Available from: http://search.ebscohost.com/login.aspx?direct=true&profile=ehost&scope=site&authtype=crawler&jrnl=16021622&AN=77706364&h=Hjcu%2B%2FuTtvQV8QNkmNtKqT0oDoeOewjDS2k2owZXQysbYELmBMRsS1ia0hZTh bM9KqG20mWEEtr1UtFRsxdKMA%3D%3D&crl=c

[18] Doerr P, Lang W, Nyquist L, Ronis D. Factors associated with dental anxiety. Journal of the American Dental Association. 1998;**129**(8):1111-1119. Available from: https://www.sciencedirect.com/science/article/pii/S0002817714662309

[19] Sohn W, Ismail AI. Regular dental visits and dental anxiety in an adult dentate population. Journal of the American Dental Association (1939). 2005;**136**(1):58-66. Available from: https://www.sciencedirect.com/science/article/pii/S0002817714655392

[20] Cohen S, Fiske J, Newton J. The impact of dental anxiety on daily living. British Dental Journal. 2000;**189**(7):385-390. Available from: https://www.nature.com/articles/4800777

[21] Folayan MO, Idehen EE, Ojo OO. The modulating effect of culture on the expression of dental anxiety in children: A literature review. International Journal of Paediatric Dentistry. 2004;**14**(4):241-245

[22] Ingman KA, Ollendick TH, Akande A. Cross-cultural aspects of fears in African children and adolescents. Behaviour Research and Therapy. 1999;**37**(4):337-345. Available from: https://www.sciencedirect.com/science/article/pii/S0005796798001089

[23] Ollendick TH, Yang B, King NJ, Dong Q, Akande A. Fears in American, Australian, Chinese, and Nigerian children and adolescents: A cross-cultural study. The Journal of Child Psychology and Psychiatry and Allied Disciplines. 1996;**37**(2):213-220. DOI: 10.1111/j.1469-7610.1996.tb01393.x

[24] Carter AE, Carter G, Boschen M, Alshwaimi E, George R. Pathways of fear and anxiety in dentistry: A review. World Journal of Clinical Cases. 2014;**2**(11):642. Available from: https://www.ncbi.nlm.nih.gov/pmc/articles/PMC4233415/

[25] Beaton L, Freeman R, Humphris G. Why are people afraid of the dentist? Observations and explanations. Medical Principles and Practice. 2014;**23**(4):295-301. Available from: https://www.karger.com/Article/Abstract/357223

[26] Hmud R, Lj W. Dental anxiety: Causes, complications and management approaches. Journal of Minimum Intervention in Dentistry. 2009;**2**(1):67-78. Available from: http://www.moderndentistrymedia.com/sept_oct2007/hmud.pdf

[27] Porritt J, Buchanan H, Hall M, Gilchrist F, Marshman Z. Assessing children's dental anxiety: A systematic review of current measures. Community Dentistry and Oral Epidemiology. 2013;**41**(2):130-142. DOI: 10.1111/j.1600-0528.2012.00740.x

[28] Dailey Y, Humphris G, Lennon M. The use of dental anxiety questionnaires: A survey of a group of UK dental practitioners. British Dental Journal. 2001;**190**(8):450-453. Available from: https://www.nature.com/articles/4801000

[29] Appukuttan D. Strategies to manage patients with dental anxiety and dental phobia: Literature review. Clinical, Cosmetic and Investigational Dentistry. 2016;**8**:35. Available from: https://www.ncbi.nlm.nih.gov/pmc/articles/PMC4790493/

[30] Humphris GM, Wong H-M, GTR L. Preliminary validation and reliability of the modified child dental anxiety scale. Psychological Reports. 1998;**83**(3_suppl):1179-1186. DOI: 10.2466/pr0.1998.83.3f.1179

[31] Humphris GM, Clarke HMM, Freeman R. Does completing a dental anxiety questionnaire increase anxiety? A randomised controlled trial with adults in general dental practice. British Dental Journal. 2006;**201**(1):33-35. Available from: https://www.nature.com/articles/4813772

[32] Hull P, Humphris G. Anxiety reduction via brief intervention in dentally anxious patients: A randomized controlled trial. Social Science and Dentistry. 2010;**1**:108-117. Available from: http://research-repository.st-andrews.ac.uk/handle/10023/2141

[33] Newton T, Asimakopoulou K, Daily B, Sclambler S, Scott S. The management of dental anxiety: Time for a sense of proportion? British Dental Journal. 2012;**213**(6):271-274. Available from: https://www.nature.com/articles/sj.bdj.2012.830.pdf?origin=ppub

[34] Caprara HJ, Eleazer PD, Barfield RD, Chavers S, Questionnaire TA. Objective measurement of patient's dental anxiety by galvanic skin reaction. Journal of Endodontics. 2003;**29**(8):493-496. Available from: https://www.sciencedirect.com/science/article/pii/S0099239905603913

[35] Skaret E, Berg E, Kvale G, Raadal M. Psychological characteristics of Norwegian adolescents reporting no likelihood of visiting a dentist in a situation with toothache. International Journal of Paediatric Dentistry. 2007;**17**(6):430-438. DOI: 10.1111/j.1365-263X.2007.00869.x

[36] Chadwick BL. Assessing the anxious patient. Dental Update. 2002;**29**(9):448-454. DOI: 10.12968/denu.2002.29.9.448

[37] Armfield J, Slade G, Spencer A. Dental fear and adult oral health in Australia. Community Dentistry and Oral Epidemiology. 2009;**37**(3):220-230

[38] Mcgrath C, Bedi R. The association between dental anxiety and oral health-related quality of life in Britain. Community Dentistry and Oral Epidemiology. 2004;**32**(1):67-72. DOI: 10.1111/j.1600-0528.2004.00119.x

[39] Kumar S, Bhargav P, Patel A, Bhati M, Balasubramanyam G, Duraiswamy P, et al. Does dental anxiety influence oral health-related quality of life? Observations from a cross-sectional study among adults in Udaipur district, India. Journal of Oral Science. 2009;**51**(2):245-254. Available from: https://www.jstage.jst.go.jp/article/josnusd/51/2/51_2_245/_article/-char/ja/

[40] Berggren U, Meynert G. Dental fear and avoidance: Causes, symptoms, and consequences. Journal of the American Dental Association. 1984;**109**(2):247-251. Available from: https://europepmc.org/abstract/med/6590605

[41] Moore R, Brødsgaard I, Rosenberg N. The contribution of embarassment to phobic dental anxiety: A qualitative research study. BMC Psychiatry. 2004;**4**(1):10-20. Available from: http://bmcpsychiatry.biomedcentral.com/articles/10.1186/1471-244X-4-10

[42] Elter J, Strauss R, Beck J. Assessing dental anxiety, dental care use and oral status in older adults. Journal of the American Dental Association. 1997;**128**(5):591-597. Available from: https://jada.ada.org/article/S0002-8177(15)60188-X/abstract

[43] Appukuttan D, Cholan P, et al. Evaluation of dental anxiety and its influence on dental visiting pattern among young adults in India: A multicentre cross sectional study. Annals of Medical and Health Sciences Research. 2017;**7**(6):393-400. Available from: https://www.amhsr.org/abstract/evaluation-of-dental-anxiety-and-its-influence-onrndental-visiting-pattern-among-young-adults-in-india-arnmulticentre-cr-4011.html

[44] Moore R, Brødsgaard I. Dentists' perceived stress and its relation to perceptions about anxious patients. Community Dentistry and Oral Epidemiology. 2001;**29**(1):73-80. DOI: 10.1034/j.1600-0528.2001.00011.x

[45] Shapiro M, Melmed RN, Sgan-Cohen HD, Eli I, Parush S. Behavioural and physiological effect of dental environment sensory adaptation on children's dental anxiety. European Journal of Oral Sciences. 2007;**115**(6):479-483. DOI: 10.1111/j.1600-0722.2007.00490.x

[46] Schneider A, Andrade J, Tanja-Dijkstra K, White M, Moles DR. The psychological cycle behind dental appointment attendance: A cross-sectional study of experiences, anticipations, and behavioral intentions. Community Dentistry and Oral Epidemiology. 2016; **44**(4):364-370. DOI: 10.1111/cdoe.12221

[47] Abrahamsson KH, Berggren U, Hallberg L, Carlsson SG. Dental phobic patients' view of dental anxiety and experiences in dental care: A qualitative study. Scandinavian Journal of Caring Sciences. 2002;**16**(2):188-196. DOI: 10.1046/j.1471-6712.2002.00083.x

[48] Crego A, Carrillo-Díaz M, Armfield JM, Romero M. From public mental health to community oral health: The impact of dental anxiety and fear on dental status. Frontiers in Public Health. 2014;**2**:16. Available from: http://journal.frontiersin.org/article/10.3389/fpubh.2014.00016/abstract

[49] Kritsidima M, Newton T, Asimakopoulou K. The effects of lavender scent on dental patient anxiety levels: A cluster randomised-controlled trial. Community Dentistry and Oral Epidemiology. 2010;**38**(1):83-87. DOI: 10.1111/j.1600-0528.2009.00511.x

Chapter 4

Anxiety as an Epileptical Equivalent (Temporal Lobe Epilepsy)

Luis A. Pando-Orellana

Additional information is available at the end of the chapter

http://dx.doi.org/10.5772/intechopen.78241

Abstract

To consider anxiety as an epileptical equivalent, several considerations have to be taken into account. First of all, what is anxiety and what is if possible a universal conception of epilepsy, and I say this because although we have the DSM series, the International League Against Epilepsy and everybody talks about "consensus" the way we classify almost every syndrome in medicine tends to dilute due to the diversity of clinical manifestations that have to be taken into account, so where and how do we apply such terms. There we have our "new" platform to understand, directly and indirectly, the role of temporal lobe syndromes, which, by the way, we all "have" but need to be discerned, as we can appreciate in EEG quantitative analysis: as to why temporal lobe is always marking for increased activity?

Keywords: anxiety, epilepsy, temporal lobe, limbic

1. Introduction

Examples of these are headaches, even though we have classic definitions and descriptions of such "disease" in Oliver Sacks in his book Migraine [1], in which, by the way, he makes a central point and establishes serious questioning toward cultural aspects of photopsias: a kind of environment influence and memory in its manifestations.

Once upon a time, during my practice in the Lacandon jungle during the late 1970s, a patient came in talking and complaining using the indigenous Mayan Tzéltal language; said to my interpreter: I feel **Kuúch, which means pain:** But what kind of pain?

The usual semiology did not work within this context. He had a **heart ache** which at the end of this consultation meant, he was depressed and the anxiety made his heart "ache."

I asked myself if this heart could really "ache" though it came from emotional impact. The answer (to my best clinical knowledge) was YES, it aches. What else could drive this man to search for help, in a context of magical thoughts, shamanes and syncretic ideas?

Years later as a specialist, I became very interested in the temporal lobe, with a very big question: is the temporal lobe and its connections with ventral-lateral thalamus responsible of such symptoms?

Again the answer was YES. And if so, how to prove it?

Again if so: can we consider the temporal lobe and its connections the real rhythm **pacer** of the brain, instead of the occipital? Again the answer is YES [2].

The quest started about 20 years ago: Prove it!

So here are the facts that were gradually published in my native language: Spanish [2–4].

www.evpol.com.mx

Reviewing antecedents and history, we owe a great deal to three persons: Paul Broca, Wilder Penfield, and Isaac Costero. We are talking a century later about the Cajal legacy from Spain.

Paul Broca a century ago talked and supported the internal brain or Limbic system, Wilder Penfield mapped the homunculus 1930s, and Costero (1980s) established the neurovegetative connections of carotid sensors with CNS and thalamic connections.

There we have our "new" platform to understand, directly and indirectly, the role of temporal lobe syndromes, which by the way we all "have" but need to be discerned, as we can appreciate in EEG quantitative analysis (**Figure 1**): as to why temporal lobe is always marking for increased activity?

So up to now, we have more data to correlate symptoms with changes in the EEG and sophisticated imaging and biological markers that do not contradict other models of Mind Brain Analysis (like the Game theory originated in the nineteenth century).

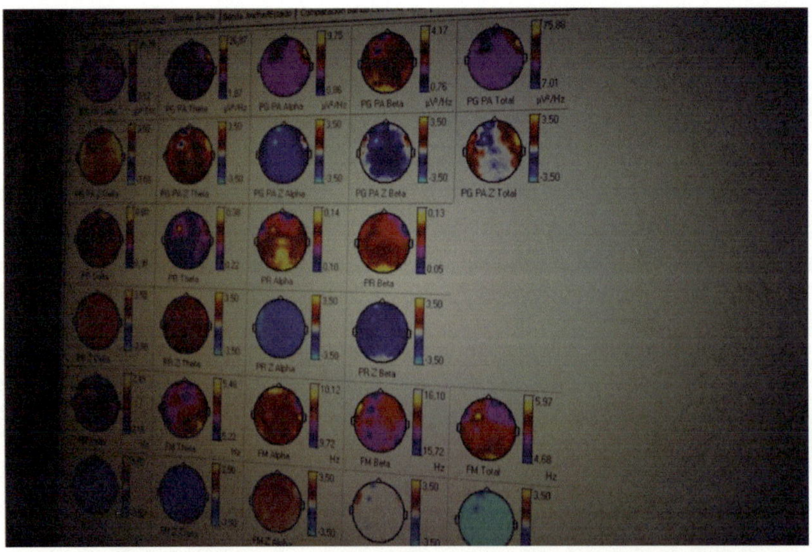

Figure 1. Geometrical power frontotemporal syndrome (courtesy of Pando et al.).

The models involve blood-brain barrier (BBB) studies of markers like S100B protein (Pando et al. in print); choline/creatine ratio visualizes through spectroscopy the affective disorders or PET/CT as marker for dementia and epilepsy particularly temporal lobe, then it has to mean something correlating it with clinical manifestations (**Figures 1–5**).

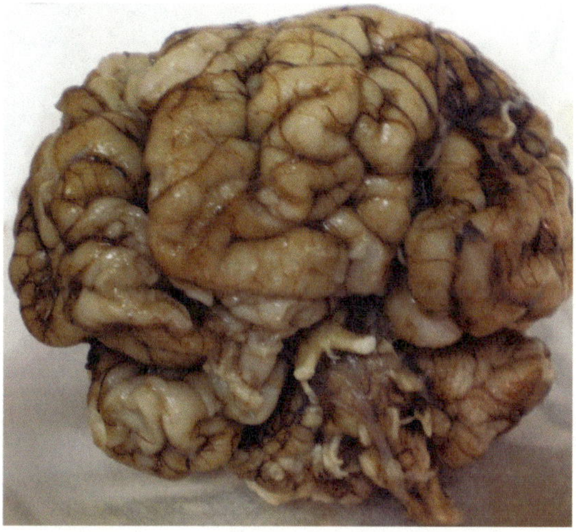

Figure 2. Frontotemporal views of one of our specimens. (courtesy of Pando et al. National institute of Cardiology "Ignacio Chavez").

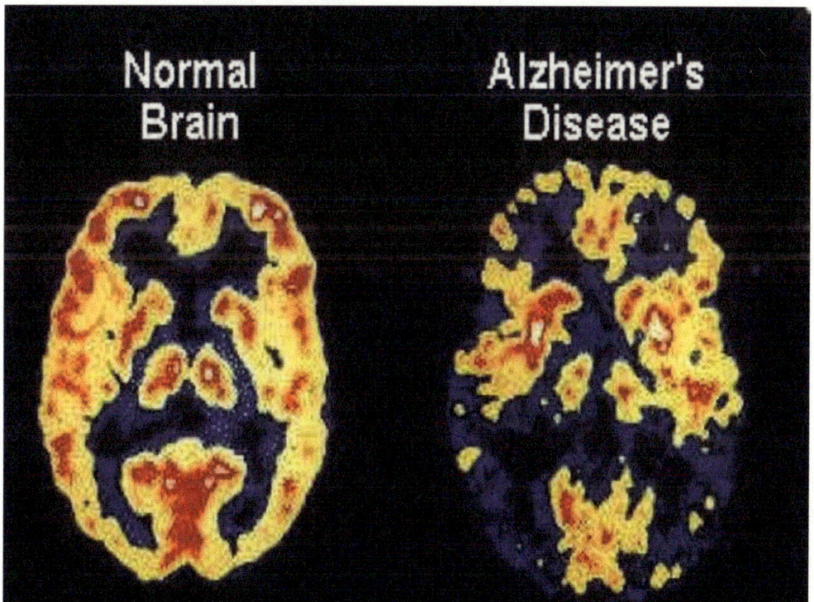

Figure 3. PET/CT with temporal lobe asymmetry (FDG marking). Courtesy of Pando et al., images from CT scanner, Mexico City.

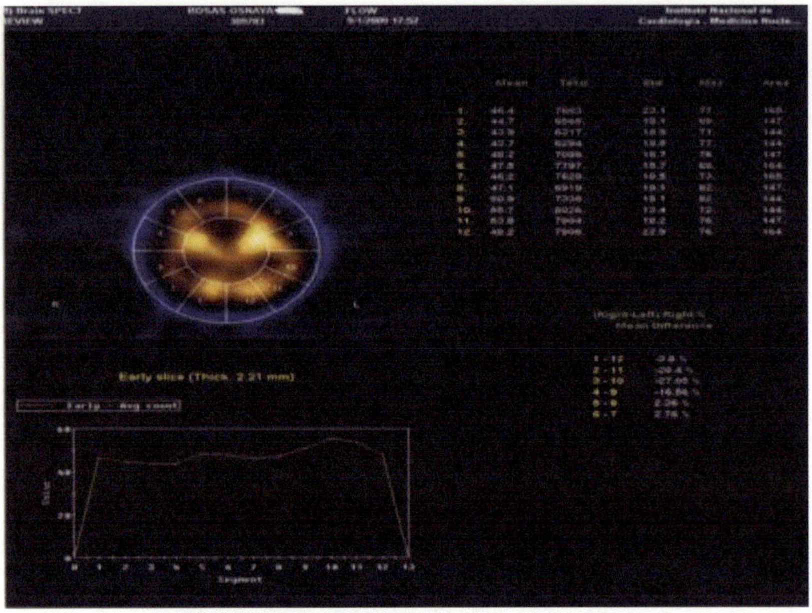

Figure 4. Single positron emitted tomography with cortical hypo-perfusion post hypovolemic shock. (Courtesy of Pando et al.).

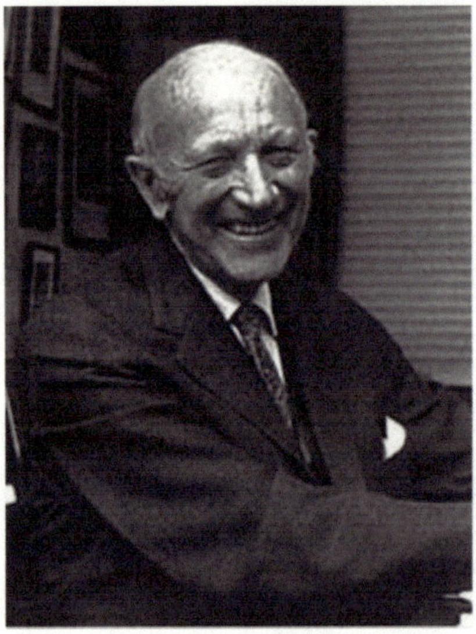

Figure 5. Wilder Penfield (public photograph). Mapped the homunculus (Johns Hopkins University).

2. Mind and game theory

These few examples of technological biomedicine can and must be applied to brain function and neuropsychiatry and not only statistics and few specialists writing "consensus" for everybody.

We all experience clinical variations of the very same frontotemporal syndrome, and these instruments are allowing us to understand how to aboard them (including autopsies) (**Figure 2**), which are being underestimated nowadays.

So if anxiety means a constant or increasing FEELING of emotional discomfort, with an urgent necessity of relief by searching just about any means available; like in the game theory, the brain responds:

If you have a certain set of cards and it is the upper hand to the "house," you pass through to the reward that is transmitting the message that your senses are sending whatever the environmental stimuli is.

There are times though in which the message does not go through, with a barrier of an overwhelmed house (brain) with demand of reward, and central temporal lobe like in medial sclerosis discharges (**Figures 1–3**), that is, with an alarm manifestation but abnormally with persistent anxiety, no matter the prefrontal cortex. So the frontal is freed from emotional filters and thought containment is surpassed within the balance that the frontal and temporal lobe must have. A psychosis is established at least for the duration of the ictus, perpetuating itself until either by internal homeorrexic mechanisms or external intervention (**Figure 2**).

The intensity of the phenomena varies from mild to panic attacks and the process can be triggered by any disrupting affective loss up to discharges that come from altered networks from a growing tumor.

Everybody "has" a frontotemporal syndrome, in any time given; [2–5] because that is how we respond emotionally; but it is to the clinician to determine the underlying pathology if so [6–11].

The temporal lobe epilepsy is one of them characterized to behave as a seizure and marking (EEG) to the temporal inferior and superior temporal gyrus [6–9, 11] (**Figure 2**).

Clinically corresponds to nine subtypes obtained through the clinical analysis and combination of temporal and frontal manifestations, considering the following variables:

C = psychotic manifestations.

P = neurodevelopmental antecedents including genetical traits.

A = epileptic behavior, including panic attacks, generalized anxiety and depressive refractory mood that fluctuates within hours.

L = individuals that simulate or plainly lie.

K = sensoperceptual dysfunction. We see what we want to see not corresponding to proper protective neural networks function and memory.

Attached a report from the EVPOL (Virtual EEG, Pando et al.) SYSTEM that correlates the geometric power of the cerebral map with a 100 question inventory of frontotemporal manifestations related as well to anxiety and panic attacks [2–5] (**Figure 6**).

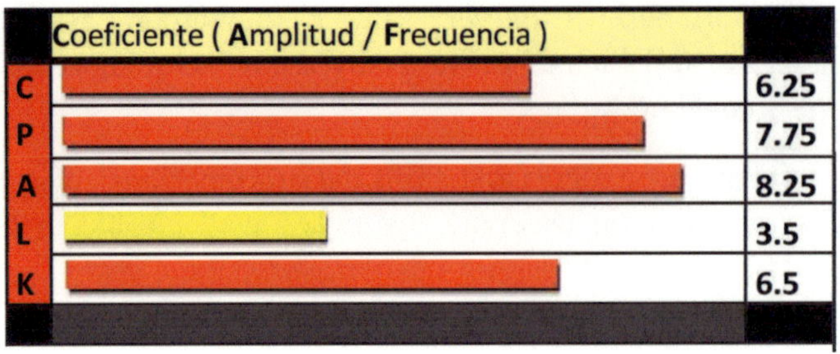

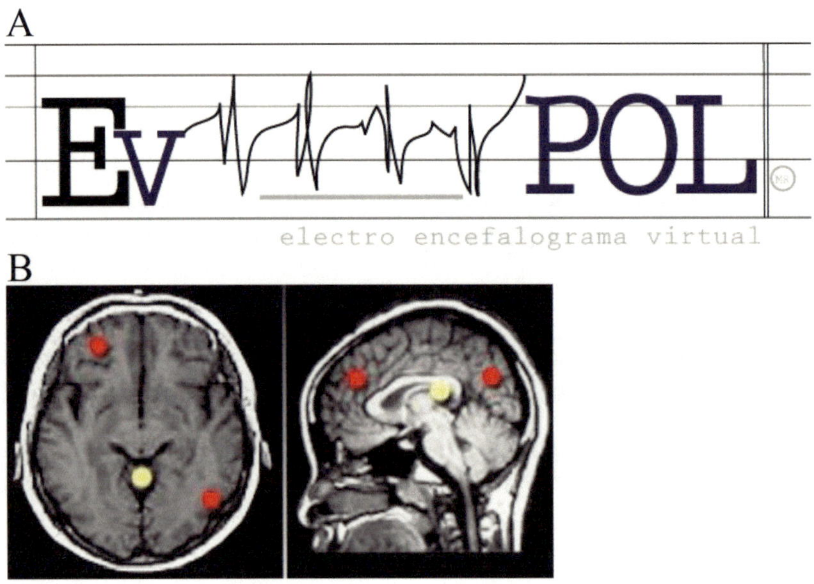

Figure 6. (A) EVPOL logo. Courtesy of Pando et al. research lab in CPALC., Mexico City. (B) MRI of brain with marking of abnormal activity. Courtesy of Pando et.al research lab in CPALC. Mexico City.

The following is described in the opinion that is shown later. The image shows the points in the brain linked to the behaviors.

- Opinion:
    - There are antecedents of risk to health, both of a genetic nature and of consequences against environmental interactions, with implications depending on the individual's predisposition to physical or psychological illness over the course of growth and development
    - Due to family history, you cannot perceive the information correctly. You may have obvious or compensated learning disorders.
- This opinion is the product of deep scientific and clinical research. Dr. Luis Pando-Orellana endorses and issues this opinion to the best of his knowledge and belief. Dr. Luis Pando-Orellana is a doctor and Doctor of Sciences with a specialty in Neuropsychiatry and Doctor in Immunology.

- Recommendation:
    - The Neuropsychiatrist recommends consulting your doctor to improve your quality of life
- This report describes behaviors that can be changed by endogenous factors [2–5].

So as in Migraines [12], we should start to deal with an unsolved classification (at least up to now) of anxiety as epileptical equivalent and it starts with: how many days should we support the patient sedated in order to substitute benzodiazepines [4] for a better neuroregulation through anticonvulsive psycho-neuropharmacology with much lesser risks of addictions or nephron-hepatic conditions with sometimes smaller doses than the ones recommended by the pharmaceutical industry [4, 6–11].

The definition of epilepsy is a paroxistic abnormal electrical discharge of any given group of neurons and any group of neurons based on the principle, one neuron, one function: networks develop through vectorial signals that are received at the level of neurofilaments which have quantic sensors in the concept of space, time, and structure that Schrodinger developed in the 30s of the past century, using Riemann tensors [2, 13].

As such if any group of given neuron discharges and recruits a network, ectopically, any given signs and symptoms should or potentially have to manifest themselves and can be registered in cuanti-qualitative analysis of the EEG and or other imaging techniques (**Figure 7**).

That is why the International League against epilepsy has not closed the door for future incorporation of such epileptic manifestations.

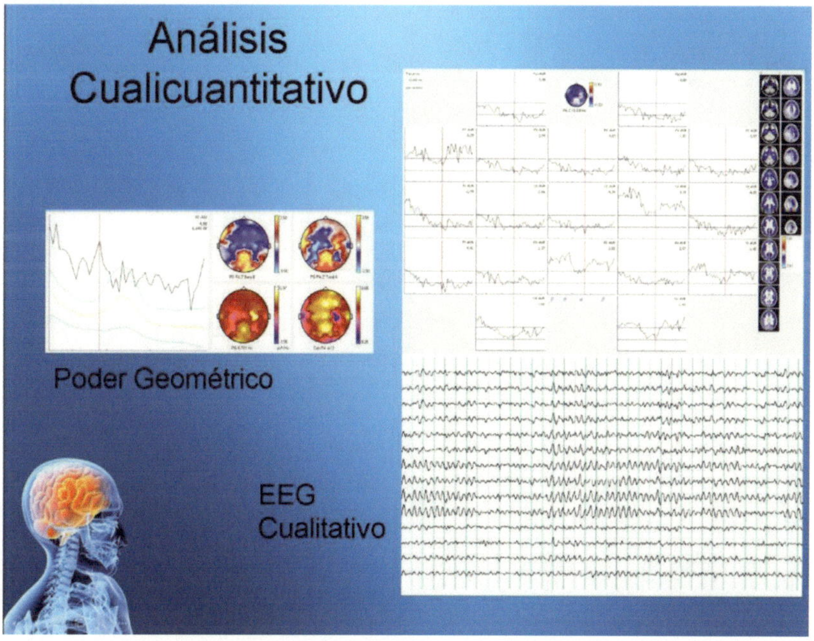

Figure 7. Quantitative analysis mapping of frontotemporal syndromes. (Courtesy of Pando et al., Mexico City).

Signals that are transcribed as semiconductors (neurofilaments) transit through synaptic trees in real time and stock these information for short periods of time between 1 ms up to more than 1 s from one membrane to another through an inter-synaptic space; the first membrane of 50 Å (thickness) initiates the process.

All the way in a tetra-dimensional quanta information traveling through tensors and counter tensors, finding their way through space networks, and respecting the thermodynamical laws with an infinitesimal delay in this essential form of computational quantic central nervous system activity [2, 13] (**Figures 7–10**).

We have worked with human models from the cuts taken during anatomic-pathological autopsies of children around 8 years of age who died from accidents (**Figure 2**).

The findings corroborate the convergence/divergence composition from the third, pyramidal neurons of the cerebral cortex. The cortex in the hypocampus shows the same composition, and we think that this is a step for recruiting neurons and to form neural networks provide the structural basis of holograms, as shown in the following sketches [2, 13] (**Figures 8–10**).

So if anxiety can be accepted as a most common form of co-morbidity or "aura" in most of structural or functional alterations of the CNS, we must also consider the probable fact that

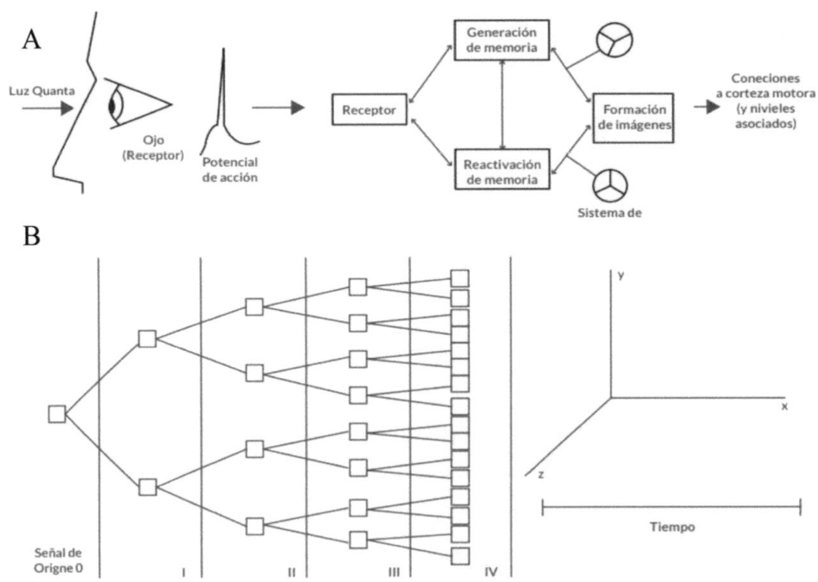

Figure 8. (A) Diagram showing the transformation of a photic stimulus and its amplification in the encephalon, generating the formation of an image and an associated memory. (Courtesy Pando et.al). (B) Diagram showing the phenomenon of amplification of information through the convergence/divergence principle in the time domain. (Courtesy Pando et al.).

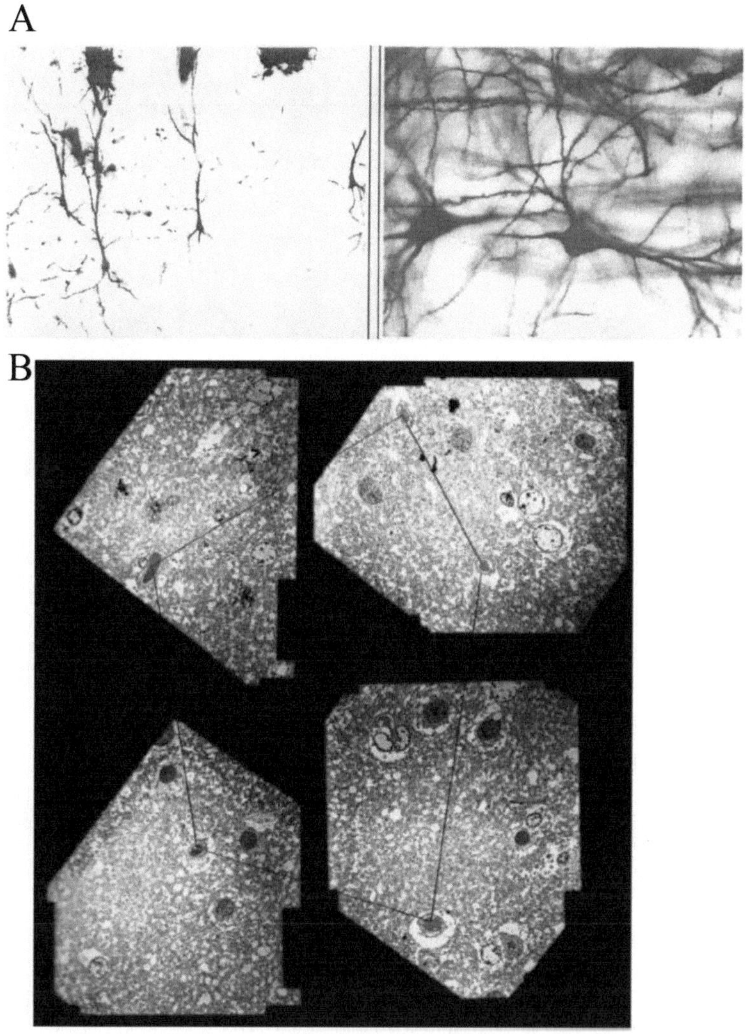

Figure 9. (A) Microphotographs with optical microscopy of cells of the primary visual cortex that were studied morphologically in the present study. Pando-et. al. Pathology Hospital Infantil de México. (Courtesy of Pando, et al.) (B) Microphotographs showing the superposed lines of the geometrical relation of the cell bodies.

within the definition of epilepsy, it can and must also be considered as an epileptical equivalent [1, 3, 4, 6–11, 13].

Mechanisms underlying pathological characteristics have yet to be fully elucidated as stated by Nemeroff et al. (2003), but since then the biochemical research regarding GABA and receptor bioengineering of drugs that block GABA receptors, thus inciting in anxiety response, particularly with gabapentine and derivates working as neuromodulators and compared to the use of benzodiacepines. This must be taken as a proof that anxiety and panic attacks [14]

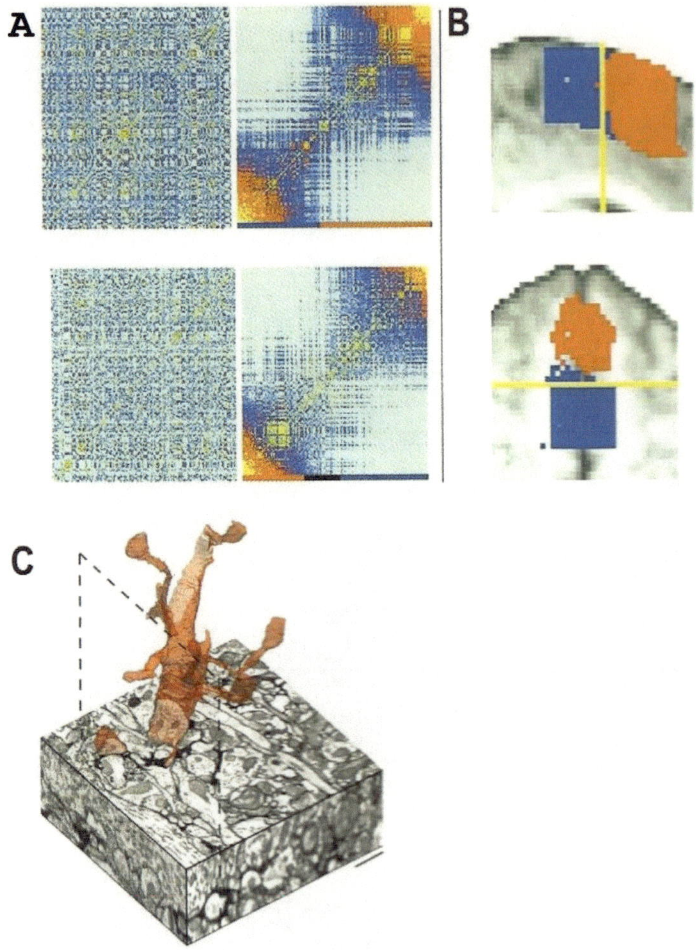

Figure 10. From bidimensional formations through fractal mathematics, we obtain images as "holograms" that are the perception of each individual during the process of each individual's perception and networks from the outside or inside world (A–C). Courtesy from Neuroradiology authored book by Stoopen M, García R. Advances in Diagnosis through Images. 2010. Journal ed. Arg. (Spanish).

as well as post-traumatic stress [1, 15–17] respond to drugs that act within the context of neuromodulation of epileptical phenomena [18] (**Figures 11–13**).

So GABA deals with phosphorylation, highly reactive for activation of mRNA and process of transcription to produce antioxidative products, regulating these proceedings through NADPH and also regulates succinate and glutamate to stabilize neurons (includes Astroglía) (Shatsberg et al. 2008; Pando et al. 2017; Doctoral thesis National Politechnical Institute, National School of Biological Science) [18].

So which drugs interact with GABA if associated to anxiety?

The answer to this question goes rapidly to anticonvulsive drugs. More than inhibitors of the recapture of serotonine, and particularly at the subcortical level in the basic ganglia [18].

http://dx.doi.org/10.5772/intechopen.78241

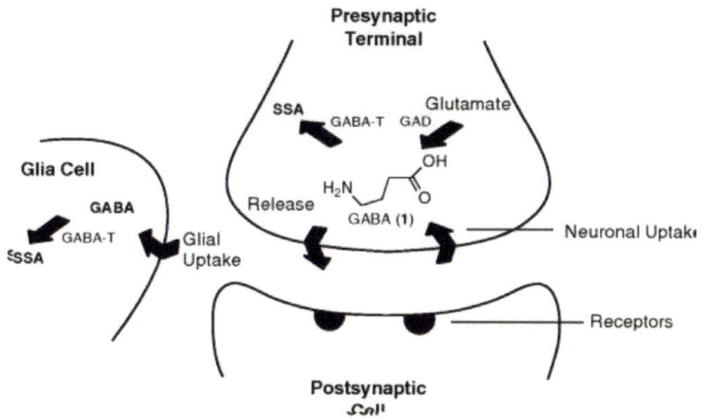

Figure 11. GABA synapsis diagram. Courtesy from Neurochemistry by Laguna et al. Biochemistry 2013, Unam, Mexico. Lehninger 6th edition and Nihon Yukirigaku, The life cycle of GABA. Faculty of Dental Science, Japan.

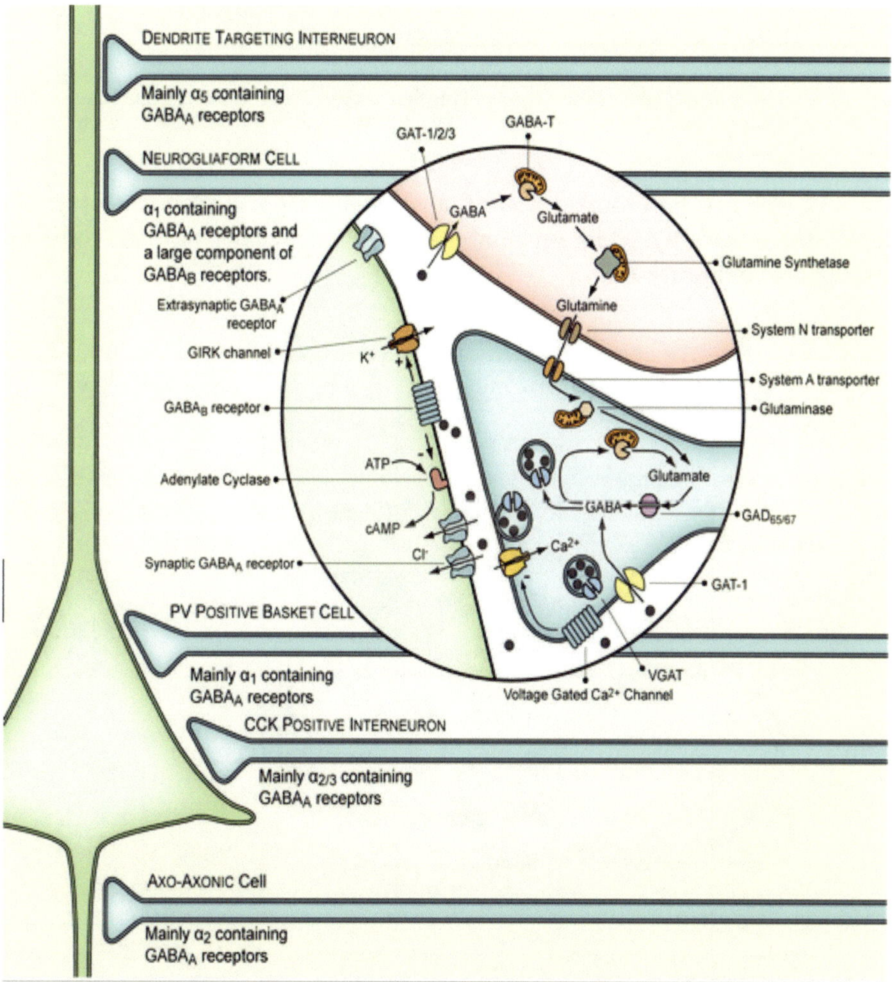

Figure 12. Drugs Associated to Gaba: Gaba receptors. Ubication of Gaba Receptors. (public scheme).

Natural Transmitter	*Selected Associated Effects*	*Interacting Psychotropic Drugs*
Acetylcholine	Learning, motor functions	Nicotine (at nicotinic sites)
Amino Acids		
Glutamate	Excitatory responses, memory, learning	Ethyl alcohol (ethanol)
GABA	Anxiety/relaxation, coordination, intoxication	Barbiturates, benzodiazepines, ethanol
Monoamines		
Dopamine	Pleasure/reward, craving, mental illness	Cocaine, amphetamines, ethanol
Norepinephrine	Stress, arousel, learning, sleep	Cocaine, amphetamines
Serotonin	Sleep, craving, mood regulation, anxiolysis	Ethanol, MDMA, hallucinogens
Neuropeptides		
Enkephalins	Pain response, learning, eating	Heroin, morphine, other opioids
Beta-Endorphins	Pain sensitivity, euphoria, pleasurable effects.	Heroin, morphine, other opioids, ethanol

Figure 13. Functions of neuromodulators. From Hospital Fray Bernardino Alvarez resident's internal operating manual, Mexico.

Antiepileptic drugs can be grouped according to their major mechanism of action. Some antiepileptic drugs work by acting on combination of channels or through some unknown mechanism of action (**Figure 14**).

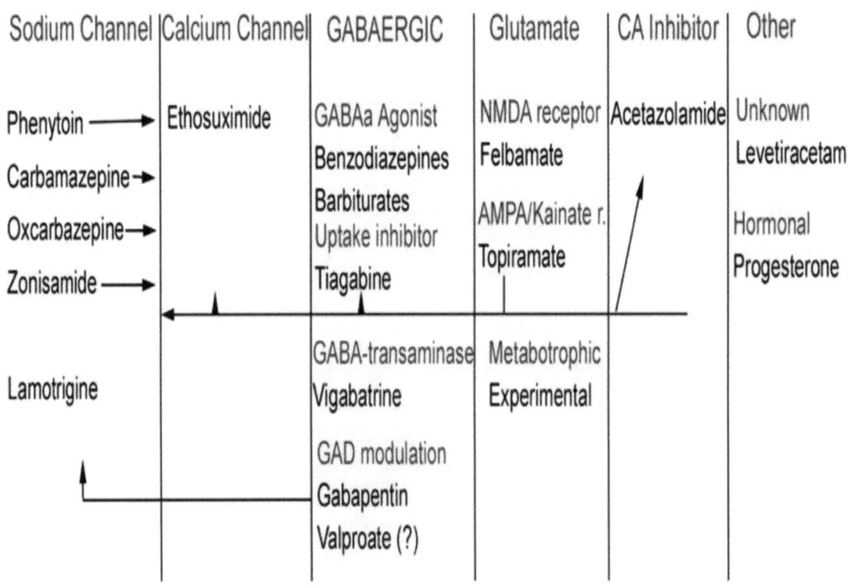

Figure 14. Drugs and site of action. (Courtesy of Fray Bernardino Alvarez Hospital).

http://dx.doi.org/10.5772/intechopen.78241

As seen, the proposition to treat anxiety with other neuromodulators, including fitopharmacology different from antidepressives or benzodiacepines, is a serious and documented stand in anxiety therapeutics [18].

Most literatures talk about anxiety, but a very few intend to define it, because it is a subjective feeling and even the DSM in any version talks about it as a comorbidity of many pathologies, but does not define it as such; the proposal is to promote anxiety as an epileptic entity; its definition as another variety of epilepsy when related to temporal lobe epilepsy or diencephalic alterations belonging to the limbic system [19–22].

Conflict of interest

There are no conflict of interests in this manuscript. The funding comes from CPALC Mexico city (Centro Para la Atención de Lesiones Cerebrales).

Author details

Luis A. Pando-Orellana

Address all correspondence to: drpando@hotmail.com

CPALC/INCIch., Mexico City, Mexico

References

[1] Torta R, Keller R, et al. Epilepsia. 1999;**40**(Suppl. 10):s2-s20

[2] Pando-orellana LA, Cabrera ML, Diaz Cintra S, et al. Modelo matemático de la relación functional neural, basado en microestructura. Revista Mexicana de Neurociencia. 2016;**17**(3):3-1

[3] Vera F, Pando-Orellana LA, et al. EEG in patients with anxiety disorder. Revista Mexicana de Neurociencia. 2013;**14**(6):335-340

[4] Pando LA. et al. Medical addictions. Revista Mexicana de Neurociencia. 2014;**15**(3):179-182

[5] Pando-Orellana LA et al. EVPOL questionnaire confiability and validity of the instrument in a sample of Mexican patients. Revista Mexicana de Neurociencia. 2009;**10**(6):443-445

[6] Johnson EK, Jones JE, Seidenberg M, Hermann BP. The relative impact of anxiety, depression, and clinical seizure features on health-related quality of life in epilepsy. Epilepsia. 2004;**45**:544-550

[7] Reuber M, Andersen B, Elger CE, Helmstaedter C. Depression and anxiety before and after temporal lobe epilepsy surgery. Seizure. 2004;**13**:129-135

[8] Park SP, Song HS, Hwang YH, Lee HW, Suh CK, Kwon SH. Differential effects of seizure control and affective symptoms on quality of life in people with epilepsy. Epilepsy & Behavior. 2010;**18**:455-459

[9] Ettinger AB, Wisbrot DM, Nolan EE, et al. Symptoms of depression and anxiety in pediatric epilepsy patients. Epilepsia. 1998;**39**(6):595-599. DOI: 10.1111/J1528-1157.1988.tb01427.X

[10] Heicemovich H, Salpekar J, Kamer AM, et al. Suicidal and epilepsy: A neuropsycho biological perspective. Epilepsy & Behavior. 2011;**22**(1):77-84. DOI: 10.1016/j.yebeh.2011.04.059

[11] Jacoby A, Snape D, Baker GA. Determinants of quality of life in people with epilepsy. Neurologic Clinics. 2009;**27**:843-863

[12] Sacks O. Migraine. USA: Random House; 1992. Collection Vintage 1999

[13] Schrödinger E. Space, Time and Structure. Cambridge Classics. Cambridge University Press; 1950. Reprint: 1985

[14] Thompson SA, Duncan JS, Smith SJM. Partial seizures presenting as panic attacks. BMJ. 2000;**321**(7267):1002-1003

[15] Markand ON, Salanova V, Whelihan E, Emsley CL. Health- related quality of life outcome in medically refractory epilepsy treated with anterior temporal lobectomy. Epilepsia. 2000;**41**:749-759

[16] Jones JE, Jackson DC, Chambers KL, et al. Children with epilepsy and anxiety: Subcortical and cortical differences. Epilepsia. 2015;**56**(2):283-290

[17] Kanner AM. Depression and epilepsy: Do glucocorticoids and glutamate explain their relationship? Current Neurology and Neuroscience Reports. 2009;**9**(4):307-312

[18] Schatzberg AF, Nemeroff CB. Textbook of Psychophamacology. 4th ed. The American Psychiatric Publishing; 2000

[19] Hamit H, Blackmon K, Cong X, et al. Mood, anxiety, seizure control affect quality of life after epilepsy surgery. Neurology. 2014;**82**(10):887-894

[20] Herman JP, Mueller NK, Figueiredo H. Role of GABA and glutamate circuitry in hypothalamic-pituitary adrenal axisdtress integration. Annals of the New York Academy of Sciences. 2006;**29**

[21] Pando-Orellana LA et al. Mental health? Revista Mexicana de Neurociencia. 2012;**13**(3): 168-169

[22] Van Campen JS, Hessel EVS, Bombach K, et al. Stress and corticoids agravate morphological changes in dentate gyrus after early life, experimental seizures in mice. Frontiers in Endocrinology (Laussane). 2018;**3**. DOI: 10.3389/fendo.2018.eCollection 2018

Chapter 5

Manifestation and Treatment of OCD and Spectrum Disorders within a Pediatric Population

Fugen Neziroglu and Yvette Fruchter

Additional information is available at the end of the chapter

http://dx.doi.org/10.5772/intechopen.79344

Abstract

The following chapter describes the presentation, impact, and treatment of obsessive compulsive disorder (OCD) in a pediatric population. Similarities and differences in the assessment and treatment of childhood-onset OCD and adult-onset OCD are noted. Children with OCD may struggle with additional mental health conditions such as anxiety, depression, and ADHD. The authors discuss the importance of addressing comorbid mental health conditions and clarify factors that may be involved in differential diagnosis. Additionally, the impact of the family environment and parent-child interactions on children with OCD is reviewed. It is common for pediatric and adult individuals with OCD to involve close family members in OCD-related behaviors in some capacity. Accommodation refers to family members' modification of their own behavior in order to assist in their child's OCD-related rituals. Addressing family accommodation in treatment can substantially impact treatment outcomes in children with OCD. Finally, evidence-based treatment modalities for pediatric obsessive compulsive disorder are explored including cognitive behavior therapy and psychiatric medication.

Keywords: OCD, pediatric, cognitive behavior therapy, family therapy, OCD medication

1. Introduction

Obsessive-compulsive disorder (OCD) has been exhibited in children as early as age 3 and all the way through adolescence and into adulthood [1]. If untreated, OCD can greatly impact children's and adolescents' abilities to thrive and participate in their lives. Functional impairment for children is frequently exhibited across various life domains including scholastic, family, social, and recreational realms [2]. Additionally, symptoms often remain or intensify as children develop. A thorough understanding of pediatric OCD symptoms and treatment recommendations can help ensure that children are appropriately screened, assessed, and provided with effective treatment and resources.

About 1–3% of children are estimated to carry an OCD diagnosis [3, 4]. Several studies have found that males are overrepresented in pediatric OCD populations, while females hold the majority in adult cases [5]. Male's age of onset of OCD tends to be between the ages of 5 and 15 years, while women have a bimodal distribution, either developing it during childhood or during pregnancy [6].

While there are many similarities between childhood-onset OCD and adult-onset OCD, several distinguishing factors are noted. Individuals with OCD onset in childhood and early adolescence are more likely to exhibit a gradual increase in symptoms and less likely to attribute triggering events, whereas individuals who develop OCD in adulthood are likely to identify possible environmental factors such as pregnancy or job loss as well as a sudden onset of symptoms [7]. Studies have also revealed individuals with early-onset OCD are likely to have a strong family history of OCD [8, 9].

Certain clinical features such as magical thinking, tapping/rubbing, and collecting compulsions as well as motor and vocal tics are more common in childhood OCD [7]. Comorbidity patterns may differ as well with children more often presenting with ADHD and tic disorders, while adults tend to present with mood-related difficulties [10]. Symptom clusters appear to manifest somewhat differently within pediatric and adult populations. Research has indicated five common symptom dimension groups in adults through factor analysis of the Yale-Brown Obsessive Compulsive Scale (YBOCS) (cleaning, symmetry, forbidden thoughts, harm, and hoarding) and about three groups in children based on Children's Yale-Brown Obsessive Compulsive Scale (harm/sexual, symmetry/hoarding, and contamination/cleaning) [11, 12].

Children may also not necessarily recognize the irrational nature of their OCD symptoms and may not describe their symptoms as distressing. Abstract thinking and hypothesis testing are still developing during childhood so the ability to draw conclusions or make connections between symptoms and restrictions on daily living is limited. In fact, a study exploring insight in 71 youths with OCD who were part of a larger treatment trial found significant differences in insight between age groups [13]. About 48% of preadolescents (ages 8–10) were categorized as high insight, while close to 72% of younger adolescents (ages 11–13) and 79% of older adolescents (ages 14–17) were categorized as high insight [13]. Thus, younger children may have a hard time addressing their symptoms due to the potential lack of understanding of the impact of OCD. Lower insight in children has been linked to greater OCD severity, higher parent-reported OCD-related impairments, and higher family accommodation [14]. A thorough assessment of insight in children is recommended; should a child appear to have poor insight, increased involvement of family members is likely warranted.

It may also be that children do not report beliefs around their compulsions, while adults do because the beliefs may be explanations adults give to their compulsions. In other words, if you have an urge to perform a particular task, you experience a feeling (e.g., anxiety) and you perform the motor act. Then you give in to the urge and try to explain why you performed a motor act. Adults usually try to explain their behaviors and have the language as well as the associations formed between certain behaviors and learned explanations, for example, we wash our hands to be clean, we look things over to be thorough and avoid mistakes, we even things up because symmetry is aesthetically pleasing, etc. It may be worth investigating at what point do children begin to explain their behaviors. As for pure obsessions, they are spontaneous thoughts over which neither children nor adults have any control except for their reaction to the thought.

2. Comorbidity

Most children who have OCD also suffer from additional mental health issues similar to their adult counterparts. Comorbidity with OCD presents considerable challenges including greater symptom severity, worse functional impairment, and poorer treatment response [2]. While studies tend to vary on percentages of comorbid conditions, they consistently demonstrate that anxiety, depression, ADHD, tic disorder, and oppositional defiant disorder are typical concerns for the pediatric OCD population [15, 16].

A recent study of 322 children with a primary diagnosis of OCD found that almost two-thirds of the sample met criteria for at least one additional diagnosis beyond OCD, with a number of comorbidities ranging up to six mental health diagnoses [16]. Only 34% of the sample presented solely with OCD. Similar to other studies, anxiety was the most common comorbidity (50%), followed by externalizing disorders including ADHD and ODD (16%), followed by depression (12%), and followed by tic disorder (11%). Adolescents (ages 14–17) in particular were most likely to have comorbid difficulties compared to preadolescents (ages 10–13) and children (ages 7–9) in particular depression, which was six times more likely [16].

Since most children who present in OCD specialty clinics will likely have co-occurring conditions, it is important that pediatric OCD assessments address the presence and impact of potential comorbidities. Decisions about treatment alterations related to comorbidities often come up as well. For example, if a child meets criteria for depression and OCD, is it necessary to have stages of treatment that address each issue separately or is it possible that CBT for OCD will address both? In fact, some studies have suggested that depressive disorders are often secondary to OCD and treating OCD as usual will typically lead to improvements in depression [15]. It is also possible that symptoms from another condition can interfere with a child's ability to absorb or tolerate therapy as usual; a child with ADHD may have trouble concentrating during sessions, whereas a child with ODD may act out during sessions. In these cases, it is particularly important to continue assessment in initial treatment stages so that any possible issues can be identified and addressed as necessary.

3. Differential diagnosis

Before discussing various disorders that need to be differentiated from OCD, it is important to recognize that within normal development there are rituals that would not be considered dysfunctional.

3.1. Normal development

Young children often seek out and find comfort in routines, for example, reading the same bedtime story every night, playing with the same toys each time at the library, or requesting the same afternoon snack every day. While these behaviors may appear ritualistic on the surface, they would not be classified as compulsions if they do not cause significant impairment or are excessively time-consuming; additionally, interruption of these rituals typically would not cause severe distress in the child [17]. Generally, children will gradually reduce their reliance and preference for these rituals as they age with little issue. These routines are to be distinguished from the presence of obsessions and compulsions, which often involve repetitive behavior, however, typically at a higher frequency and intensity and with the addition of high anxiety and distress when rituals are interrupted. Notably, children do not customarily just "grow out" of OCD so it is important that parents address the issue and provide appropriate treatment rather than minimize the impact of the symptoms or accommodate as a short-term fix [18, 19].

3.2. When do rituals become dysfunctional?

Obsessive compulsive disorder involves intrusive and anxiety-provoking thoughts, images, and/or impulses (obsessions) and repetitive mental or behavioral actions intended to reduce anxiety and prevent feared negative consequences (compulsions), which cause distress, are time consuming, and cause functional impairment [20]. The content of obsessions and compulsions often varies such that OCD can appear quite heterogeneous across cases: one child may repeatedly wash their hands throughout the day in an effort to prevent life-threatening illnesses, while another child repeats certain phrases to ensure "bad" thoughts do not lead to the occurrence of "bad" events. Additionally, two children may wash hands repeatedly and display similar compulsions for entirely different obsessional themes (for example, one child may fear germs, whereas another child seeks a "just right" feeling). The Children's Yale-Brown Obsessive Compulsive Scale (CY-BOCS) is considered the gold standard for assessment of OCD and includes a clinician-rated checklist of common obsessions and compulsions, which allows for specificity and clarity of symptoms [21].

Diagnosing OCD is complicated as it manifests quite differently across cases and symptoms can appear similar to other disorders [22]. Children and adolescents may attempt to hide their symptoms due to shame or embarrassment about having "bad" or irrational thoughts or unusual behaviors, which may cause parents or clinicians to miss or overlook dysfunction [17]. As children are still developing with regard to verbal communication abilities, they may not articulate clear obsessions. Similarly, mental rituals may go undetected. Also, as discussed above, children with OCD may have comorbid conditions, which can lead to challenges in distinguishing symptoms between diagnoses. Symptoms of different conditions can look quite similar in presentation; that is, does a child who repeatedly asks for reassurance and checks for physical ailments related to fear of throwing up have a separate phobia or is the fear of vomiting considered another manifestation of OCD? Certain tics can also manifest quite similarly to behavioral compulsions related to symmetry or "just right" feeling. Differential diagnosis must be carefully conducted particularly in situations where treatment recommendations would differ. Below are some disorders that need to be considered in differential diagnosis.

http://dx.doi.org/10.5772/intechopen.79344

3.3. PANDAS/PANS

"Pediatric autoimmune neuropsychiatric disorders associated with streptococcal infections" (PANDAS) refers to a particular subtype of pediatric OCD with abrupt onset, episodic course of illness, and a number of distinctive features [23, 24]. The original diagnostic criteria for PANDAS included (1) the presence of OCD and/or a tic disorder, (2) onset of these symptoms prior to puberty, (3) abrupt onset of symptoms, and (4) association with autoimmune infection group A streptococcus (GAS) [24]. The autoimmune response in PANDAS contributes to inflammation of the basal ganglia and subsequent dysfunction of the brain structure [24]. Researchers began investigating PANDAS when they identified a subset of pediatric individuals who had an unusual course of OCD symptoms: a sudden dramatic onset followed by a gradual reduction over several months [23, 24]. They noted similarities to individuals with Sydenham's chorea (a type of rheumatic fever) and, upon further investigation, noted that numerous patients with chorea also had obsessive compulsive symptoms as well.

PANDAS symptoms are documented as early as age 3 and intensification of symptoms can occur within mere days [24]. An investigation of 50 clinical case studies identified average age of onset for PANDAS with obsessive compulsive symptoms at 7.4 and with tic symptoms at 6.3 [24]. To be classified as PANDAS, the symptoms must be temporally related to GAS infection such as a positive throat culture or elevated anti-GAS antibody titers. Patients also often exhibit neurological irregularities such as motor hyperactivity and tics though these may wax and wane during periods of remission. Other symptoms associated with PANDAS include impulsivity, distractibility, emotional lability, separation anxiety, age-inappropriate behavior, bedwetting, and handwriting disabilities [24, 25]. Of note, PANDAS-like symptoms have been exhibited in response to other bacterial and viral infections including influenza, varicella, mycoplasma infections, and chronic Lyme disease [26].

Recently, researchers noted potential challenges with the original diagnostic criteria of PANDAS (such as difficulty establishing temporal association with GAS infection as well as difficulty distinguishing between PANDAS and non-PANDAS cases). Thus, researchers have reviewed the original diagnostic criteria and available data to establish PANS: pediatric acute-onset neuropsychiatric syndrome [26]. PANDAS is now considered under the rubric of PANS. Diagnostic criteria for PANS include (1) abrupt, dramatic onset of obsessive compulsive disorder, (2) severely restricted food intake, (3) concurrent presence of additional neuropsychiatric symptoms from at least two of the following seven categories: anxiety; emotional lability and/or depression; irritability or aggression; behavioral regression; reduced school performance; motor abnormalities; somatic symptoms including sleep disturbance, enuresis, or urinary frequency, and (4) symptoms are not better explained by a neurological or medical disorder [26]. PANS is conceptualized as a broader clinical entity that can be related to a preceding infection; however, it also refers to acute-onset symptoms without apparent immune disturbance [26]. If a child does exhibit the clinical criteria of PANS, the possibility of PANDAS should be explored and appropriate laboratory studies conducted to determine any association to GAS or other infectious triggers.

Treatment for PANS includes standard OCD treatments including exposure and response prevention as well as psychotropic medications (selective serotonin reuptake inhibitors,

SSRIs) [27]. Additional treatment options specific to PANDAS that are being explored include antibiotics, tonsillectomy, nonsteroidal anti-inflammatory drugs (NSAIDS), therapeutic plasma exchange (TPE), intravenous immunoglobulin (IVIG), and anti-CD20 monoclonal antibodies (rituximab) [27].

3.4. Generalized anxiety disorder

A child who has difficulty controlling worries about everyday issues would likely be exhibiting symptoms of generalized anxiety disorder (GAD). GAD involves excessive worry about real-life concerns, while OCD centers on irrational fears that are unrealistic and beyond the scope of daily life problems [22, 28]. At times, these disorders can be clearly distinguished, for example, when one child worries excessively about an upcoming math test while another is overwhelmingly concerned about receiving a deadly illness from germs or turning into an animal by the power of their thoughts. Sometimes, however, the differential diagnosis may be less clear-cut; for example, a child's concern about his mother flying on an airplane could be categorized as a worry about his mother's well-being (GAD) or irrational fear of harm toward loved ones (OCD). Furthermore, pathological worry may function similarly to mental compulsions as both are self-initiated and aimed at reducing distress [28]. It has been suggested that compulsions can be distinguished from pathological worry by its frequency (compulsions will likely have a higher number of repetitions), rigidity (a child with OCD is more likely to seek the same answer over and over, whereas a child with GAD may ask numerous questions about different risks), quality (compulsions are likely to be more illogical such as tapping an object repeatedly to prevent harm to a loved one), and function (compulsions for OCD often seek to reduce distress related to thought of future negative events, whereas pathological worry seeks to reduce occurrence of future negative event but as no compulsions or acts involved in preventing the outcome) [28].

3.5. Tic disorders

Tics refer to sudden, repetitive, stereotyped movements or sounds. While tics are often perceived as involuntary, they usually are accompanied by premonitory sensory urges [29]. Simple tics include eye blinking, neck jerking, shoulder shrugging, or throat clearing. Complex tics can involve facial gestures, touching, smelling objects, or repeating words or phrases; often complex tics involve repeating certain actions until it feels right. Simple tics are more easily distinguished from compulsions due to their brevity, lack of purpose, and seemingly involuntary nature, while complex tics can present quite similarly to compulsions [29]. A behavior that functions to reduce distress or anxiety (e.g., repeatedly tapping the sidewalk to prevent a feared consequence) is likely to be related to OCD, while a behavior that functions to relieve somatic discomfort or tension (e.g., repeatedly moving arm in certain way in response to discomfort) [22]. Additionally, clinicians can ask if withholding the behavior would result in anxiety or physical discomfort. Looking at the symptom in context of the child's history can be helpful as well depending on if the child has presented with anxiety and/or distinct obsessions or compulsions vs. simple tics with minimal anxiety [22].

3.6. Autism

Individuals with autism spectrum disorders often display rigid interests and repetitive behaviors, which can appear similar to obsessions and compulsions. Common repetitive behaviors associated with autism disorder include repetitive motor mannerisms, preference for sameness, distressing reactions to change, and perseveration on a restricted range of interests [30]. It has been suggested that repetitive behavior in autism is a source of pleasure rather than a reaction to anxiety [30]. Querying about developmental history may help differentiate between OCD and autism such as screening for history of language delays and difficulties with social interactions. Additionally, fixed interests in autism are typically experienced as ego-syntonic and even enjoyable, while symptoms in OCD are often distressing and experienced as ego-dystonic [22].

3.7. Eating disorder

Patients with eating disorders (EDs), similar to OCD, experience intrusive thoughts that contribute to maintenance of dysfunctional behaviors. Intrusive thoughts in ED typically center on food, diet, physical exercise, and appearance [31]. These intrusions trigger negative affect, which leads to engagement in behaviors to alleviate discomfort such as checking weight, compulsive exercise, binge eating, purging, or restricting food intake. Thus, both ED and OCD involve intrusive thoughts related to feared negative outcomes, which are linked to compensatory behaviors intended to reduce emotional distress [31]. OCD can present similarly to ED (for example, severe weight loss from contamination-focused OCD due to fears that food is dirty); eating only certain foods that are perceived to keep in good health for those with health-related OCD. Also the reverse can be true where patients with ED may appear to be OCD; for example, avoid having oils around due to fear of contamination of the food with fats; counting the number of bites of a piece of food; cutting the food into a certain number of pieces, etc. Studies that have assessed frequency of obsessions and compulsions in OCD and ED (particularly anorexia nervosa) patients have found symmetry obsessions and ordering compulsions to be most common for ED, while OCD patients tend to have more variety of symptoms [32].

3.8. Primary vs. secondary depression

Depression is often comorbid with OCD and may be treated differently whether it is secondary and occurring in response to the stress caused by OCD or it is a primary condition that is separate from the OCD. Comorbid depression is associated with increased OCD symptom severity and increased functional impairment [14, 33]. Screening for depression is important to ensure treatment is effective and taking into account a person's overall well-being. Notably, several studies have revealed that treating OCD through exposure and response prevention can lead to a decrease in comorbid depression and that treatment outcomes are not worsened by the presence of depression [15, 34, 35]. Distinguishing whether depression is primary or secondary to OCD can guide treatment decisions whether to begin with exposure and response prevention or to begin with CBT targeting depression. Assessing the content of depressive cognitions can provide information on whether depressive thoughts center on impairment or quality of life issues related to OCD. Additionally, obtaining a timeline of symptoms (such as whether depression preceded OCD or began afterward) can assist with identifying if depression is reactionary to OCD or a distinct condition.

4. Course of the disorder

While OCD has frequently been described as a debilitating and chronic illness whose symptoms wax and wane over time, less is known about the course of the disorder for children and adolescents specifically. In fact, research demonstrates potential differences regarding the course of illness between pediatric and adult populations. A study that compared pediatric and adult treatment-seeking individuals with OCD over a 3-year time period found that children had a significantly higher remission rate (53%) compared to adults (34%) [36]. Better psychosocial functioning as well as engaging in treatment earlier in the course of illness was related to shorter time to remission for children with OCD. These findings suggest a better prognosis for pediatric OCD and additionally emphasize the importance of early recognition and intervention for children with OCD [36].

Additionally, clinical presentation of OCD may vary across the life span between children, adolescents, and adults. Youth diagnosed with OCD at an earlier age tend to have higher rates of ADHD and anxiety disorders [1, 37]. As children with OCD age into adolescence, they are more likely to experience mood disorders such as depression [1, 16, 37]. These developmental trends are exemplified by a study that investigated differences in clinical presentation between 46 children, 55 adolescents, and 60 adults with OCD. Results revealed that ADHD and tic disorder rates were inversely related to age such that the children had the highest prevalence followed by adolescents and then adults [37]. Conversely, adults had the highest rates of depression followed by adolescents and then children with the lowest rates of depression [37]. Similarly, another study that examined the prevalence of comorbidity in pediatric OCD demonstrated adolescents had a six times greater likelihood of having a co-occurring depressive disorder compared to younger children [16].

5. Etiology

OCD pathogenesis involves neuroanatomy, biochemical, genetic, and environmental factors. Brain structures that are associated with obsessive compulsive disorder include the orbitofrontal cortex, striatum, thalamus, and the basal ganglia, which are all involved in the cortical-striatal circuit [38]. MRI and fMRI scans have demonstrated structural abnormalities for individuals with OCD. Biochemical factors that have been identified to play a role include neurotransmitters like serotonin [38, 39], and in fact, serotonin changes have been shown to change purely with an intensive exposure and response prevention treatment [40]. Genetic factors also appear to have a strong influence on the development of early-onset OCD. Children

http://dx.doi.org/10.5772/intechopen.79344

with OCD are likely to have other first-degree relatives that also have OCD as well as anxiety, mood, ADHD, and tic disorders [9]. Numerous studies have demonstrated elevated rates of OCD in parents of children with early onset of the disorder, including a study that found a quarter of fathers and almost 10% of mothers meeting criteria for OCD [41]. For a subset of individuals, the pathogenesis of OCD is related to an autoimmune infectious disease known as autoimmune neuropsychiatric disorders associated with Streptococcus (PANDAS), which is also implicated in Tourette's disorder. It has been suggested this year that PANDAS be renamed to encephalitis autoimmune disorder poststreptococci.

With regard to environmental factors, family environment has been identified as a likely contributor to OCD development in children [42]. Social learning is theorized to play an important role in the development of childhood anxiety disorders. Children learn from seeing how their parents function in the world and how their parents cope with their own anxiety and emotional distress. Additionally, parent communication style and relationship quality impacts child development of psychopathology. Authoritarian parenting style (low warmth, high behavioral control) has been linked to higher incidences of obsessive compulsive symptoms and obsessive compulsive beliefs (such as regarding the importance of thoughts and personal responsibility) [43]. This finding is consistent with other studies that have demonstrated an association between parental control and higher rates of child anxiety [44]. Family factors are therefore important to address in the treatment of pediatric OCD.

6. Parent-child interactions

Children's OCD symptoms affect and are affected by family dynamics and the family environment. As children are heavily reliant on their parents for activities of daily living and general well-being, parents often bear the brunt of their child's OCD severity and impairment. Extensive research demonstrates the importance of accounting for family factors in the treatment of pediatric OCD [45–48]. In fact, family-based therapy has demonstrated effectiveness and is highly encouraged, especially in the case of younger children [45, 49].

A parent of a child with OCD is faced with many challenges on a daily basis. Children may delay family activities due to involvement in rituals or may refuse to partake in activities or gatherings altogether due to their OCD symptoms. When children become distressed by their obsessions and compulsions, it is typically family members who deal with the resulting temper tantrums, crying, reassurance seeking, or avoidance of situations and activities. Children may request or demand their parents adjust their behavior to assist with rituals or prevent feared negative consequences related to obsessional fears (e.g., expecting a parent to hand-wash excessively after a parent touches something the child considers dirty). Parents are faced with difficult questions such as how to cope effectively with their children's emotional distress, whether to assist in rituals or provide reassurance, and how to respond when children avoid or refuse to participate in activities. In addition, parents often have to deal with the poor interpersonal relations these children exhibit [50].

6.1. Pediatric OCD and family accommodation

A child, age 8, becomes tearful after accidentally touching something in a public area due to worries of becoming severely ill. She cries and asks her mother repeatedly "Am I going to be sick and die?" The child's mother answers the question, "No, that's not possible, you aren't going to become sick from that"; however, the girl appears unsatisfied and continues to ask similar questions. When her mother eventually tells her she already answered the question and attempts to end the conversation, the daughter throws herself onto the floor and begs her mother to answer again. The mother knows from past experience that when she answers her daughter, she is likely to calm down sooner and experience relief. However, she has also observed that her daughter seems to ask more frequently for reassurance and seems to want her mother to repeat the answer more times. What is this mother's best choice in this situation?

It is common for pediatric and adult individuals with OCD to involve close family members in OCD-related behaviors in some capacity [51, 52]. Accommodation refers to family members' modification of their own behavior in order to assist in their child's OCD-related rituals [53–55]. This may occur in a variety of forms including participating in rituals themselves (e.g., washing their hands excessively at their child's request or listening to repeated confessions of their child), facilitating avoidance of situations (e.g., picking child up early from school or removing knives in home if child has aggressive obsessions), and providing reassurance (e.g., saying nothing bad is going to happen in response to child asking about a harm-related fear).

Research suggests that the majority of families engage in accommodation on a regular basis. An analysis of the Pediatric OCD Treatment Study (POTS) explored the prevalence of family accommodation as well as whether there are child or parent factors that are related to a tendency toward accommodation. The POTS is a randomized controlled trial that investigated the effectiveness of cognitive behavioral therapy alone, medication alone, and the combination of therapy and medication, compared to a placebo control condition in children (ages 7–17) with OCD and their families [56]. In a subset of 96 individuals who completed the Family Accommodation Scale Parent Report (FAS-PR), 99% of parents reported engaging in at least one accommodating behavior to some extent and 77.1% reported engaging in at least one accommodating behavior daily [53]. More than half of parents reassured their child (63.5%), while about a third participated in their child's OCD rituals (32.33%) and assisted in avoiding triggering situations (33.3%) on a daily basis [53]. These results are comparable to other studies that have explored the prevalence of accommodation in pediatric OCD [46, 57].

Parents typically accommodate with their child's best interests at heart in hopes of alleviating distress, assisting with management of OCD symptoms, and/or improving family functioning. Accommodation often does result in short-term relief and can appear helpful when, for example, a child ceases tantruming after receiving reassurance. In reality, OCD symptoms are actually maintained as rituals are negatively reinforced and the child learns they cannot handle their fears without compulsions. Family accommodation has been shown to be associated with symptom severity pretreatment for children and adolescents with OCD, further evidence that this practice actually worsens rather than solves the problem [46, 57, 58]. Yet, children eventually come to expect family participation in rituals and become agitated when family members attempt to change the system. Thus, parents can often feel powerless to intervene and feel compelled to continue accommodation even if they realize it may exacerbate symptoms over time.

In an effort to understanding the family processes that contribute to accommodation, researchers have explored the correlates and predictors of this phenomenon. Within the 96 families involved in the POTS cited above, more severe rituals, oppositional behavior, and higher frequency of washing symptoms in children contributed to increased parental accommodation. Parental anxiety was also identified as a relevant factor, which suggests that as parents' anxiety increases, they may have a harder time setting boundaries and disengaging from requests to participate in rituals [53]. A study of 65 children and their families (ages 8–17) also demonstrated that child symptom severity as well as parent anxiety, parent hostility, and parent psychopathology correlate with accommodation. Additionally, higher family conflict was associated with more accommodation-related distress and worse consequences when not accommodating while higher family organization was associated with the less accommodation-related distress [57]. Thus, without addressing family or parent-related factors, cognitive behavioral therapy can be compromised and lead to less beneficial outcomes. A prospective, longitudinal study found that parental accommodation (measured at intake) was the strongest predictor of OCD symptom severity at intake and 2-year follow-up, again demonstrating the impact of family factors on pediatric OCD [54]. This study analyzed data from an ongoing, prospective study, the Brown Longitudinal Obsessive Compulsive Disorder Study (BROWNS), to examine the predictive value of parental accommodation (assessed at intake) on OCD symptom severity at intake and 2 years after intake after controlling for factors such as child age, anxiety, and depression [59]. Results revealed, as discussed above, that parental accommodation at a single point in time may have a strong influence on predicting future OCD symptom severity. Potentially, family accommodation patterns become so entrenched that they are maintained over time due to the potential short-term effects of sudden accommodation changes (child becoming agitated and expressing distress). Thus, unless intervention directly targets family factors, one may expect parental accommodation to remain a strong predictor of future OCD symptoms and outcome.

Addressing family accommodation in treatment can substantially impact treatment outcomes in children with OCD [46, 58]. In a study of 50 youth and families who participated in family-based cognitive behavioral therapy, family accommodation was common among the participants and was associated with symptom severity before treatment [46]. Decreases in family accommodation during treatment predicted treatment outcome even when controlling for pretreatment OCD severity. Accordingly, treatment protocols for OCD are increasingly emphasizing reduction of family accommodation as an important therapeutic factor.

7. Assessment practice guidelines

The 2012 evidence-based practice parameters published by the American Academy of Child Adolescent Psychiatry detail assessment recommendations for pediatric OCD symptoms [17].

Routine screening of obsessions and compulsions is recommended during all psychiatric evaluations of children and adolescents, regardless of whether OCD is part of the presenting complaint. Screening can be conducted via several brief questions such as "Do you have worries that just won't go away or get stuck" and "Do you do things over and over or have habits you can't stop?" [17]. For individuals who exhibit OCD symptoms and meet DSM criteria for the disorder, a comprehensive evaluation of possible comorbid psychiatric disorders is recommended as well as a thorough medical, developmental, family, and school history [17]. As discussed in comorbidity section above, children are likely to present with multiple diagnoses, which may impact their treatment needs and ability to participate effectively in OCD treatment. With regard to family history, inquiries should focus on family mental health history, activities of daily living, general family dynamics, and lifestyle factors. Medical history questions may also provide helpful information regarding differential diagnosis of PANDAS/PANS. Additionally, gathering information about a child's academic performance over time also allows for an understanding of functional impairment and symptom severity outside of the child's home [17].

8. Treatment practice guidelines

Evidence-based treatment modalities for pediatric obsessive compulsive disorder comprise cognitive behavior therapy (CBT), specifically exposure and response prevention (ERP), as well as psychiatric medication (selective serotonin reuptake inhibitors, SSRIs) [17, 45, 60, 61]. CBT is recommended as the first-line treatment for mild-to-moderate cases of OCD in children [17]. A combination of psychotropic medication and CBT is recommended for moderate-to-severe OCD in children, with serotonin reuptake inhibitors considered the first-line medication [62]. Additionally, medication can be helpful in cases where children are having difficulties engaging in treatment or have co-occurring disorders that cause additional functional impairment. Medication augmentation may also be considered for individuals with treatment resistance (i.e., nonresponsive to empirically based interventions) who experience persistent OCD symptoms despite adequate treatment interventions.

9. Cognitive behavioral therapy for pediatric OCD

Exposure and response prevention (ERP) involves prolonged, repeated contact with feared stimuli that trigger obsessions (exposure) without engagement in compulsive or avoidant behaviors (ritual prevention) [63, 64]. Treatment will usually start with psychoeducation to orient the child and family to the cognitive behavioral model and expectations for therapy. The therapist, child, and often family members will then collaborate to create a list of situations that trigger anxiety and rate them from lowest to highest intensity (i.e., treatment hierarchy). Exposures will typically begin with situations that trigger mild anxiety and proceed in a graded fashion as the child habituates (experiences a reduction in anxiety) and/or increases their willingness to remain in the situations despite anxiety. Simultaneously, the child does not engage in rituals before, during, or after exposure to block negative reinforcement and to allow the anxiety to decline naturally. For example, a child who worries about contracting a serious illness and engages in excessive handwashing and avoidance of germs would not only touch objects that are associated with germs but also refrain from handwashing for the exposure exercise.

9.1. Family involvement in treatment

Family-based CBT programs have been recommended for early childhood OCD (approximately ages 5–8) and have demonstrated success in randomized control trials [45, 61]. Parent participation is particularly important for younger children who have unique developmental needs and rely heavily on their caretakers. The Pediatric Obsessive-Compulsive Disorder Treatment Study for Young Children (POTS JR) evaluated the efficacy of a family-based CBT protocol (FB-CBT) for young children who addressed cognitive, socioemotional, and family factors compared to a family-based relaxation training protocol [45]. This 14-week randomized clinical trial involved 127 pediatric outpatients with OCD aged 5–8 years at three academic medical centers. Results revealed that the FB-CBT led to significant reductions in OCD symptoms and functional impairment; young children with OCD were able to benefit from exposure and response prevention with parental support [45].

Family-based CBT incorporates parent tools such as behavior management skills training; parents are trained in behavioral strategies such as implementing reward systems, modeling, and ignoring behaviors that are reinforced by attention [45]. As children may lack insight into their symptoms and/or resist voluntary contact with triggers, they may be more likely to participate in treatment with the addition of external reinforcers. Additionally, parents can be actively involved during in-session and home-based exposure exercises and provide helpful support to their child. Therapists teach parents how to act as a coach between sessions, which ensures increased likelihood of children practicing and adhering to CBT principles between sessions [45]. Parents who are included in the treatment process are less likely to accommodate their child's OCD, which can greatly enhance treatment outcomes [14].

9.2. Treatment intensity

While outpatient therapy often involves a weekly schedule, the possibility of more intensive treatment can be considered depending on the child's clinical presentation and circumstances. Studies have demonstrated that daily sessions offer comparable results to weekly sessions and even provide slight advantages immediately posttreatment though there appear to be no group differences at later follow-ups [48, 49]. While weekly treatment allows for children to maintain their routines and remain in school and other activities, intensive treatment can also be considered as an option when children have a limited time frame and/or require a faster response rate. Many of our children receive intensive treatment during holidays or during the summer months. In addition, children who are unable to attend school may be considered for intensive outpatient programs.

9.3. Additional consideration for ERP in child populations

Children are encouraged to externalize the OCD as separate from themselves [64, 65]. Therapists often describe OCD as a "bully" or "worry monster" that puts "silly worries" or "scary thoughts" into the children and "commands" or "bullies" the children to repeat certain behaviors. Children externalize their OCD by giving their OCD a name of their choice (e.g., Mr. Wrong, Meanie, Silly Sam, etc.) and "bossing back" or fighting OCD by not listening to its commands and doing the opposite of what OCD says (i.e., exposures).

Psychoeducation can involve using examples from other areas of the child's life to build motivation for facing fears as a way of overcoming them (e.g., learning to ride a bike or swim). Depending on child's age or developmental level, therapists may measure level of anxiety in a variety of ways: a fear thermometer or using objects of different sizes that symbolize anxiety levels (e.g., three cups of different sizes). When possible and applicable, therapists can make exposure into a game (e.g., doing silly things in the presence of feared trigger, who can touch the dirty pen first, passing a pen between their toes and race with the therapist) to increase children's willingness to participate and match their developmental level. Additionally, including parents in the "game" or exposure activity may help children feel more comfortable and open to engage.

10. Addressing treatment obstacles and future directions

Factors associated with poorer treatment response in children with OCD include lower insight, higher family accommodation, comorbid disorders, and greater symptom severity [48, 49, 61]. Researchers are exploring ways to improve the efficacy and accessibility of OCD treatments. Potentially, strategies aimed at enhancing readiness in children may facilitate increased engagement in therapy such as motivational interviewing strategies [66]. In fact, a pilot study explored the usefulness of adjunctive motivational interviewing sessions (MI) compared to adjunctive psychoeducation sessions; results indicated the MI condition led to faster reduction in symptoms (though scores posttreatment were not significantly different from the control condition), and on average, treatment was completed three sessions earlier than those in the control group [46]. Incorporating technology may allow CBT researchers and clinicians to reach a wider audience of individuals who otherwise may not have access to treatment due to location and other logistics (e.g., childcare for other siblings, transportation availability). One pilot study found significant treatment outcomes for a web-based CBT intervention, leading to the suggestion that web-based CBT may be considered in cases where in-person sessions are not feasible [67]. Additionally, as discussed above in prior sections, family members are increasingly being included and targeted in standard CBT therapy protocols for children with OCD with substantially positive outcomes [46, 58].

Author details

Fugen Neziroglu* and Yvette Fruchter

*Address all correspondence to: neziroglu@gmail.com

Bio-Behavioral Institute, Great Neck, NY, USA

References

[1] Garcia AM, Freeman JB, Himle MB, Berman NC, Ogata AK, Ng J, et al. Phenomenology of early childhood onset obsessive compulsive disorder. Journal of Psychopathology and Behavioral Assessment. 2009;**31**(2):104-111

[2] Piacentini J, Bergman RL, Keller M, McCracken J. Functional impairment in children and adolescents with obsessive-compulsive disorder. Journal of Child and Adolescent Psychopharmacology. 2003;**13**(2, Supplement 1):61-69

[3] Flament MF, Whitaker A, Rapoport JL, Davies M, Berg CZ, Kalikow K, et al. Obsessive compulsive disorder in adolescence: An epidemiological study. Journal of the American Academy of Child & Adolescent Psychiatry. 1988;**27**(6):764-771

[4] Heyman I, Fombonne E, Simmons H, Ford T, Meltzer H, Goodman R. Prevalence of obsessive-compulsive disorder in the British nationwide survey of child mental health. International Review of Psychiatry. 2003;**15**(1-2):178-184

[5] Castle DJ, Deale A, Marks IM. Gender differences in obsessive compulsive disorder. Australian & New Zealand Journal of Psychiatry. 1995;**29**(1):114-117

[6] Neziroglu F, Anemone R, Yaryura-Tobias JA. Onset of obsessive-compulsive disorder in pregnancy. American Journal of Psychiatry. 1992;**149**(7):947-950

[7] Millet B, Kochman F, Gallarda T, Krebs MO, Demonfaucon F, Barrot I, et al. Phenomenological and comorbid features associated in obsessive–compulsive disorder: Influence of age of onset. Journal of Affective Disorders. 2004;**79**(1):241-246

[8] Nestadt G, Samuels J, Riddle M, Bienvenu OJ, Liang KY, LaBuda M, et al. A family study of obsessive-compulsive disorder. Archives of General Psychiatry. 2000;**57**(4):358-363

[9] Walitza S, Wendland JR, Gruenblatt E, Warnke A, Sontag TA, Tucha O, et al. Genetics of early-onset obsessive–compulsive disorder. European Child & Adolescent Psychiatry. 2010;**19**(3):227-235

[10] Kalra SK, Swedo SE. Children with obsessive-compulsive disorder: Are they just "little adults"? The Journal of Clinical Investigation. 2009;**119**(4):737-746

[11] Højgaard DRMA, Mortensen EL, Ivarsson T, Hybel K, Skarphedinsson G, Nissen JB, et al. Structure and clinical correlates of obsessive–compulsive symptoms in a large sample of children and adolescents: A factor analytic study across five nations. European Child & Adolescent Psychiatry. 2017;**26**(3):281-291

[12] Hybel KA, Mortensen EL, Højgaard DR, Lambek R, Thomsen PH. Symptom profiles and executive function in childhood obsessive-compulsive disorder. Journal of Obsessive-Compulsive and Related Disorders. 2017;**14**:36-46

[13] Lewin AB, Bergman RL, Peris TS, Chang S, McCracken JT, Piacentini J. Correlates of insight among youth with obsessive-compulsive disorder. Journal of Child Psychology and Psychiatry. 2010;**51**(5):603-611

[14] Storch EA, Merlo LJ, Larson MJ, Geffken GR, Lehmkuhl HD, Jacob ML, et al. Impact of comorbidity on cognitive-behavioral therapy response in pediatric obsessive-compulsive disorder. Journal of the American Academy of Child & Adolescent Psychiatry. 2008;**47**(5):583-592

[15] Brown HM, Lester KJ, Jassi A, Heyman I, Krebs G. Paediatric obsessive-compulsive disorder and depressive symptoms: Clinical correlates and CBT treatment outcomes. Journal of Abnormal Child Psychology. 2015;**43**(5):933-942

[16] Peris TS, Rozenman M, Bergman RL, Chang S, O'Neill J, Piacentini J. Developmental and clinical predictors of comorbidity for youth with obsessive compulsive disorder. Journal of Psychiatric Research. 2017;**93**:72-78

[17] Geller DA, March J. Practice parameter for the assessment and treatment of children and adolescents with obsessive-compulsive disorder. Journal of the American Academy of Child & Adolescent Psychiatry. 2012;**51**(1):98-113

[18] Abramowitz JS, Whiteside SP, Deacon BJ. The effectiveness of treatment for pediatric obsessive-compulsive disorder: A meta-analysis. Behavior Therapy. 2005;**36**(1):55-63

[19] Bloch MH, Craiglow BG, Landeros-Weisenberger A, Dombrowski PA, Panza KE, Peterson BS, et al. Predictors of early adult outcomes in pediatric-onset obsessive-compulsive disorder. Pediatrics. 2009;**124**(4):1085-1093

[20] American Psychiatric Association. Diagnostic and Statistical Manual of Mental Disorders (DSM-5). Washington, D.C.: American Psychiatric Pub; 2013

[21] Scahill L, Riddle MA, McSwiggin-Hardin M, Ort SI, King RA, Goodman WK, et al. Children's Yale-Brown obsessive compulsive scale: Reliability and validity. Journal of the American Academy of Child & Adolescent Psychiatry. 1997;**36**(6):844-852

[22] Lewin AB, Piacentini J. Evidence-based assessment of child obsessive compulsive disorder: Recommendations for clinical practice and treatment research. Child Youth Care Forum. 2010;**39**(2):73-89

[23] Allen AJ, Leonard HL, Swedo SE. Case study: A new infection-triggered, autoimmune subtype of pediatric OCD and Tourette's syndrome. Journal of the American Academy of Child & Adolescent Psychiatry. 1995;**34**(3):307-311

[24] Swedo SE, Leonard HL, Garvey M, Mittleman B, Allen AJ, Perlmutter S, et al. Pediatric autoimmune neuropsychiatric disorders associated with streptococcal infections: Clinical description of the first 50 cases. American Journal of Psychiatry. 1998;**155**(2): 264-271

[25] Orefici G, Cardona F, Cox CJ, Cunningham MW. Pediatric autoimmune neuropsychiatric disorders associated with streptococcal infections (PANDAS). In: Streptococcus pyogenes: Basic Biology to Clinical Manifestations. Oklahoma City, Oklahoma: University of Oklahoma Health Sciences Center. 2016. pp. 1-43

[26] Swedo SE, Leckman JF, Rose NR. From research subgroup to clinical syndrome: Modifying the PANDAS criteria to describe PANS (pediatric acute-onset neuropsychiatric syndrome). Pediatric Therapeutics. 2012;**2**(2):113

[27] Sigra S, Hesselmark E, Bejerot S. Treatment of PANDAS and PANS: A systematic review. Neuroscience & Biobehavioral Reviews. 2018;**86**:51-65

[28] Comer JS, Kendall PC, Franklin ME, Hudson JL, Pimentel SS. Obsessing/worrying about the overlap between obsessive–compulsive disorder and generalized anxiety disorder in youth. Clinical Psychology Review. 2004;**24**(6):663-683

[29] Mansueto CS, Keuler DJ. Tic or compulsion? It's Tourettic OCD. Behavior Modification. 2005;**29**(5):784-799

[30] Zandt F, Prior M, Kyrios M. Repetitive behaviour in children with high functioning autism and obsessive compulsive disorder. Journal of Autism and Developmental Disorders. 2007;**37**(2):251-259

[31] García-Soriano G, Roncero M, Perpiñá C, Belloch A. Intrusive thoughts in obsessive–compulsive disorder and eating disorder patients: A differential analysis. European Eating Disorders Review. 2014;**22**(3):191-199

[32] Phillips KA, Kaye WH. The relationship of body dysmorphic disorder and eating disorders to obsessive-compulsive disorder. CNS Spectrums. 2007;**12**(5):347-358

[33] Canavera KE, Ollendick TH, May JTE, Pincus DB. Clinical correlates of comorbid obsessive–compulsive disorder and depression in youth. Child Psychiatry & Human Development. 2010;**41**(6):583-594

[34] Abramowitz JS, Foa EB. Does comorbid major depressive disorder influence outcome of exposure and response prevention for OCD? Behavior Therapy. 2000;**31**(4):795-800

[35] Storch EA, Björgvinsson T, Riemann B, Lewin AB, Morales MJ, Murphy TK. Factors associated with poor response in cognitive-behavioral therapy for pediatric obsessive-compulsive disorder. Bulletin of the Menninger Clinic. 2010a;**74**(2):167-185

[36] Mancebo MC, Boisseau CL, Garnaat SL, Eisen JL, Greenberg BD, Sibrava NJ, et al. Long-term course of pediatric obsessive–compulsive disorder: 3 years of prospective follow-up. Comprehensive Psychiatry. 2014;**55**(7):1498-1504

[37] Geller DA, Biederman J, Faraone SV, Bellordre CA, Kim GS, Hagermoser L, et al. Disentangling chronological age from age of onset in children and adolescents with obsessive–compulsive disorder. The International Journal of Neuropsychopharmacology. 2001;**4**(2):169-178

[38] Lewin AB, Storch EA, Geffken GR, Goodman WK, Murphy TK. A neuropsychiatric review of pediatric obsessive-compulsive disorder: Etiology and efficacious treatments. Neuropsychiatric Disease and Treatment. 2006;**2**(1):21

[39] Yaryura-Tobias JY, Neziroglu F, Bhagavan HN. Obsessive-compulsive disorders: A serotonergic hypothesis. In: Neuro-Psychopharmacology. Vienna: Proceedings of the 11th Congress of the Collegium Internationale Neuro-Psychopharmacologicum. 1979. pp. 117-125

[40] Neziroglu F, Steele J, Yaryura-Tobias JA, Hitri A, Diamond B. Effect of behavior therapy on serotonin level in obsessive compulsive disorder. In: Stefanis CN, Rabavilas AD, Soldator CR, editors. Psychiatry: A World Perspective. Vol. 3. Amsterdam, Netherlands: Elsevier Science Publishers; 1990. pp. 707-710

[41] Lenane MC, Swedo SE, Leonard H, Pauls DL, Sceery W, Rapoport JL. Psychiatric disorders in first degree relatives of children and adolescents with obsessive compulsive disorder. Journal of the American Academy of Child & Adolescent Psychiatry. 1990;**29**(3): 407-412

[42] Grisham JR, Anderson TM, Sachdev PS. Genetic and environmental influences on obsessive-compulsive disorder. European Archives of Psychiatry and Clinical Neuroscience. 2008;**258**(2):107-116

[43] Timpano KR, Keough ME, Mahaffey B, Schmidt NB, Abramowitz J. Parenting and obsessive compulsive symptoms: Implications of authoritarian parenting. Journal of Cognitive Psychotherapy. 2010;**24**(3):151-164

[44] Ballash N, Leyfer O, Buckley AF, Woodruff-Borden J. Parental control in the etiology of anxiety. Clinical Child and Family Psychology Review. 2006;**9**(2):113-133

[45] Freeman J, Sapyta J, Garcia A, Compton S, Khanna M, Flessner C, et al. Family-based treatment of early childhood obsessive-compulsive disorder: The Pediatric Obsessive-Compulsive Disorder Treatment Study for Young Children (POTS Jr)—A randomized clinical trial. JAMA Psychiatry. 2014;**71**(6):689-698

[46] Merlo LJ, Lehmkuhl HD, Geffken GR, Storch EA. Decreased family accommodation associated with improved therapy outcome in pediatric obsessive–compulsive disorder. Journal of Consulting and Clinical Psychology. 2009;**77**(2):355

[47] Peris TS, Sugar CA, Bergman RL, Chang S, Langley A, Piacentini J. Family factors predict treatment outcome for pediatric obsessive-compulsive disorder. Journal of Consulting and Clinical Psychology. 2012;**80**(2):255

[48] Storch EA, Geffken GR, Merlo LJ, Jacob ML, Murphy TK, Goodman WK, et al. Family accommodation in pediatric obsessive–compulsive disorder. Journal of Clinical Child and Adolescent Psychology. 2007;**36**(2):207-216

[49] Storch EA, Geffken GR, Merlo LJ, Mann G, Duke D, Munson M, et al. Family-based cognitive-behavioral therapy for pediatric obsessive-compulsive disorder: Comparison of intensive and weekly approaches. Journal of the American Academy of Child & Adolescent Psychiatry. 2007;**46**(4):469-478

[50] Borda T, Feinstein BA, Neziroglu F, Vessia T, Perez-Rivera R. Are children with obsessive-compulsive disorder at risk for problematic peer relationships? Journal of Obsessive-Compulsive and Related Disorders. 2013;**2**(4):359-365

[51] Gomes JB, Van Noppen B, Pato M, Braga DT, Meyer E, Bortoncello CF, et al. Patient and family factors associated with family accommodation in obsessive–compulsive disorder. Psychiatry and Clinical Neurosciences. 2014;**68**(8):621-630

[52] Van Noppen B, Steketee G. Testing a conceptual model of patient and family predictors of obsessive compulsive disorder (OCD) symptoms. Behaviour Research and Therapy. 2009;**47**(1):18-25

[53] Flessner CA, Freeman JB, Sapyta J, Garcia A, Franklin ME, March JS, et al. Predictors of parental accommodation in pediatric obsessive-compulsive disorder: Findings from the Pediatric Obsessive-Compulsive Disorder Treatment Study (POTS) trial. Journal of the American Academy of Child & Adolescent Psychiatry. 2011;**50**(7):716-725

[54] Francazio SK, Flessner CA, Boisseau CL, Sibrava NJ, Mancebo MC, Eisen JL, et al. Parental accommodation predicts symptom severity at long-term follow-up in children with obsessive–compulsive disorder: A preliminary investigation. Journal of Child and Family Studies. 2016;**25**(8):2562-2570

[55] Storch EA, Larson MJ, Muroff J, Caporino N, Geller D, Reid JM, et al. Predictors of functional impairment in pediatric obsessive-compulsive disorder. Journal of Anxiety Disorders. 2010b;**24**(2):275-283

[56] Pediatric OCD Treatment Study (POTS) Team. Cognitive-behavior therapy, sertraline, and their combination for children and adolescents with obsessive-compulsive disorder: The pediatric OCD treatment study (POTS) randomized controlled trial. JAMA. 2004;**292**:1969-1976

[57] Peris TS, Bergman RL, Langley A, Chang S, Mccracken JT, Piacentini J. Correlates of accommodation of pediatric obsessive-compulsive disorder: Parent, child, and family characteristics. Journal of the American Academy of Child & Adolescent Psychiatry. 2008;**47**(10):1173-1181

[58] Lebowitz ER, Panza KE, Bloch MH. Family accommodation in obsessive-compulsive and anxiety disorders: A five-year update. Expert Review of Neurotherapeutics. 2016;**16**(1): 45-53

[59] Pinto A, Mancebo MC, Eisen JL, Pagano ME, Rasmussen SA. The Brown Longitudinal Obsessive Compulsive Study: Clinical features and symptoms of the sample at intake. The Journal of Clinical Psychiatry. 2006;**67**(5):703

[60] Franklin M, Foa E, March JS. The pediatric obsessive-compulsive disorder treatment study: Rationale, design, and methods. Journal of Child and Adolescent Psychopharmacology. 2003;**13**(2, Supplement 1):39-51

[61] Franklin ME, Kratz HE, Freeman JB, Ivarsson T, Heyman I, Sookman D, et al. Cognitive-behavioral therapy for pediatric obsessive-compulsive disorder: Empirical review and clinical recommendations. Psychiatry Research. 2015;**227**(1):78-92

[62] Geller DA, Biederman J, Stewart SE, Mullin B, Martin A, Spencer T, et al. Which SSRI? A meta-analysis of pharmacotherapy trials in pediatric obsessive-compulsive disorder. American Journal of Psychiatry. 2003;**160**(11):1919-1928

[63] Foa EB, Kozak MJ. Psychological treatment for obsessive-compulsive disorder. In: Mavissakalian MR, Prien RF, editors. Long-Term Treatments of Anxiety Disorders. Washington, DC: American Psychiatric Press; 1996. pp. 285-309

[64] March JS, Mulle K. OCD in Children and Adolescents: A Cognitive-behavioral Treatment Manual. New York: Guilford Press; 1998

[65] Wagner AP. Cognitive-behavioral therapy for children and adolescents with obsessive-compulsive disorder. In: Hudak R, Dougherty D, editors. Clinical Obsessive-Compulsive Disorders in Adults and Children. Cambridge: Cambridge University Press; 2011. pp. 138-151

[66] Rollnick S, Miller WR. What is motivational interviewing? Behavioural and Cognitive Psychotherapy. 1995;**23**(4):325-334

[67] Storch EA, Caporino NE, Morgan JR, Lewin AB, Rojas A, Brauer L, et al. Preliminary investigation of web-camera delivered cognitive-behavioral therapy for youth with obsessive-compulsive disorder. Psychiatry Research. 2011;**189**(3):407-412

Section 4

Stigma In Anxiety Disorders

Chapter 6

Stigma in Obsessive Compulsive Disorder

Gokcen Akyurek, Kubra Sahadet Sezer,
Leyla Kaya and Kezban Temucin

Additional information is available at the end of the chapter

http://dx.doi.org/10.5772/intechopen.83642

Abstract

Stigmatizing attitudes and behaviors of the society can be associated with avoidance of treatment-seeking behaviors and reduced quality of life for the individual with mental illness. Among these problems, individuals with mental impairment are exposed to unfair behavior in the criminal justice system, restrictions on social facilities, and most importantly, reduced their roles in their life and community participation. Although researches have gone far to understand the impact of the disease, it has only recently begun to explain stigma in mental illness. Much yet needs to be done to fully understand the breadth and scope of prejudice against people with mental illness. Therefore, this chapter presents the stigmatization and its historical development and types and stigma in mental health and obsessive-compulsive disorders to provide a brief overview of issues in the area. Moreover, this chapter presents the occupational therapy interventions in stigma both in adults and children with obsessive compulsive disorder.

Keywords: community participation, mental disorders, obsessive compulsive disorder, stigma, society

1. Introduction

Individuals with mental impairment are struggling not only with the problems caused by their illnesses but also with the stigmatizing attitudes and behaviors of the society; even for this reason, stigmatization is often referred to as "second disease" [1]. When the stigmatizing attitude of the society is accepted and internalized as it is by the stigmatized individual, the problems in the individual's life are increasing exponentially [2]. Among these problems, individuals with mental impairment are exposed to unfair behavior in the criminal justice system [3], restrictions on social facilities [4–7], and most importantly, avoidance of treatment seeking behaviors and reduced quality of life [8–10]. In addition, it is suggested that the stigmatization not only affects the lives of the members of the family and their immediate surroundings but also the quality of life [11, 12]. One of the psychiatric disorders that are exposed to such stigmatizing attitudes and behaviors is obsessive compulsive disorder (OCD) although the stigmatization effect on the individuals who have received the diagnosis of schizophrenic disorder in the first and most recent years is discussed. OCD is a chronic mental disorder that negatively affects the quality of life and social, academic, and occupational functioning of individuals and families with this disorder [13]. Obsessions and compulsions experienced by an individual with OCD diagnosis, especially the distress experienced by them, cause the individual to be more isolated from the society. Moreover, it is stated that the quality of life is affected at a similar level to the diagnosis of schizophrenic disorder in OCD diagnosis [14]. In this chapter, it was aimed to explain the effect of the stigmatization in OCD.

The problems brought by individual and familial problems with a psychiatric diagnosis already have a very negative effect. In addition, individuals with mental disorders are exclusively excluded from society because of the reactions they are likely to exhibit and possibly display, as well as other people's feelings, thoughts, and behaviors, with causal attributions, as seen in people with certain characteristics; rather than seeking treatment, they can choose to hide their problems at home and live a relatively isolated life. This, in turn, reduces the likelihood that many people with a diagnosis of being diagnosed have the potential to get treatment and solve their problems; this situation leads to many types of loss in terms of individual and society. For this reason, reducing the stigmatizing attitudes and behaviors in the society is at least as important as the treatment. In recent years, it appears that the number and nature of initiatives undertaken to reduce the stigmatization of mental disorders has increased significantly [15].

2. What is stigma?

Stigma is defined as a characteristic or disorder that separates the individual from "normal" people in society and marks them as "unacceptable." Stigma is defined by the World Health Organization [WHO] as "a sign of embarrassment, embarrassment, or rejection that has been excluded from rejection, discrimination and participation in different areas of the society." [16]. The stigmatization process involves the identification of the separating state and then the step of disqualification of the individual [17]. The purpose of the stamp is to separate and exclude the individual from society [18]. Stigma means "scar, trail, sign," but today, it is mostly used as "black spot." The stamp is considered a symptom of a situation that is to be embarrassed for a person or a group or an unusual, unacceptable sign [18]. Stigmatizing is the individual's mental or physical disability, his race, drug addiction, or any illness that is considered bad by the society. The individual is stained, flawed, and reduced to the eye of others. This causes the stigmatized individuals to fear the society and isolate itself from society [19] (**Figure 1**).

2.1. Historical development of stigma

Stigma was originally used by the Ancient Greeks and symbolizes the physical signs that one has unusual and negative qualities in social or moral status. These signs are made by

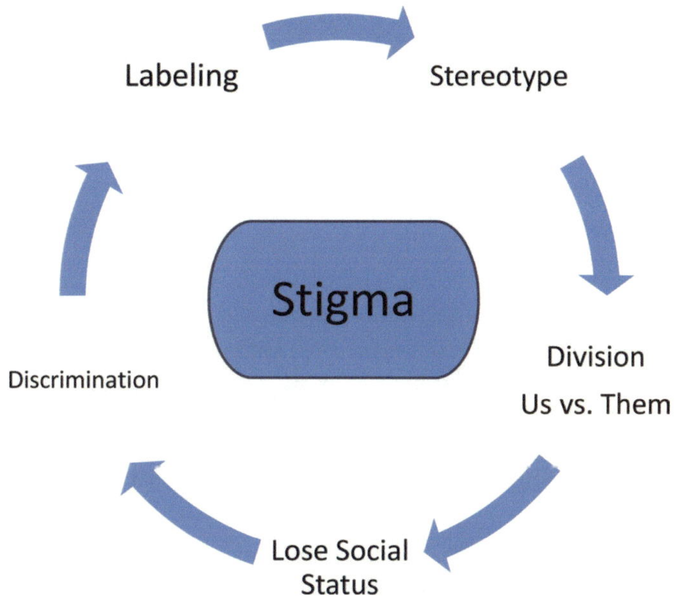

Figure 1. Problematic stigma cycle.

excavating the body or by tattooing, and evidence that a person carrying such a sign is a slave, a person who must be kept away like a criminal or a traitor. With the spread of Christianity, the term stigma is added. This ironic version refers to signs believed to have manifested itself in the form of bud-like sores on the skin, believed to be the physical signs of God's mercy, as it is in the prophet Jesus, and thus believed to be sacred. The first person to take this issue in scientific terms is Goffman [20]. Goffman describes three distinct types of content that are quite different in content: (a) differences in personality (mental disorders, homosexuality, alcoholism, addiction, imprisonment, depersonalization, etc.), (b) various physical deformations (weak wills, extreme passions, perverted and rigid beliefs and immorality, stay, unemployment, suicide attempts) and (c) ethnological stamps (race, nation and religion). Stigmatization is defined as the perception of the individual as imperfect or obtrusive rather than normal; the stigmatized individual is less valued and these people are almost not perceived as human [20]. Stigmatizing is not a new phenomenon, but the traces are based on a rather old history. Many diseases arising from the existence of mankind have been perceived as catastrophic in the society and have caused the sufferers to suffer persecution. The plague that emerged in the 1300s was regarded as a punishment sent by God to sinful people, and people with plague were declared criminals. Individuals caught up in syphilis, which is quite common in Europe during the 15th century, have been cursed for centuries. Although such specimens now seem very out of date and old, similar misconceptions and beliefs still exist today. AIDS, previously known as homosexual disease, has been considered a divine punishment given to sinful people by God [21]. As a result, stigmatization has a history as old as human history, and many diseases have been subjected to stigmatization; it continues to stay.

2.2. Types of stigma

There are several categories of stigmatization in our society, and beyond any description, stigmatization has been decisive for negative experiences at both macro and micro level. The three main types of Stigma include social stamping, self-stamping, and professional stamping (**Figure 2**). Social stigmatization is the most common.

2.2.1. Social stigma

According to Merriam Webster, social stigmatization indicates that (or dissatisfaction with) a person or group that is perceived by the other members of a society and serving to distinguish them is socially unapproved. Social theorists view such a stigma as particularly effective. A social group of the past is dependent on social information structures learned by most members [22–24]. In American society, there is a distinction between physical illness and mental illness and is based on the misperception that mental illness is a result of having a weak character or making a heretical choice [25, 26]. Social stigma against mental illness rests on this misperception [27]. This differentiation, which affects consumers, stakeholders, and providers, contributes to division and allows social stigmatization against mental illness, resulting in discrimination in diagnosis, treatment, and social perception. As a result of this social paradigm, people with symptoms are less likely to accept mental illness and receive appropriate mental health care [25–27].

Individuals are generally determined by their behavior, and unfortunately, behavioral problems associated with mental disorders result in poor self-esteem, limited participation, and reduced treatment. In addition, mental health results in avoidance of participation in services [22]. One of the difficulties of social stigmatization is that people who think that others perceive themselves differently perceive themselves differently. It is likely that the self may be stigmatized [23]. Considering that stigma is a social structure, culture significantly influences stigmatization. Culture expresses common behaviors, beliefs, values orientations, and symbols that affect a group of people's own norms and practices. These sociocultural norms and practices also define the meaning, practice, and expression of the stigmatization in different populations [28, 29].

2.2.2. Self-stigmatization

According to the literature, self-stigma is associated with perceived stigma. Persons suffering from mental illness will become self-imposed when they acknowledge that the people are

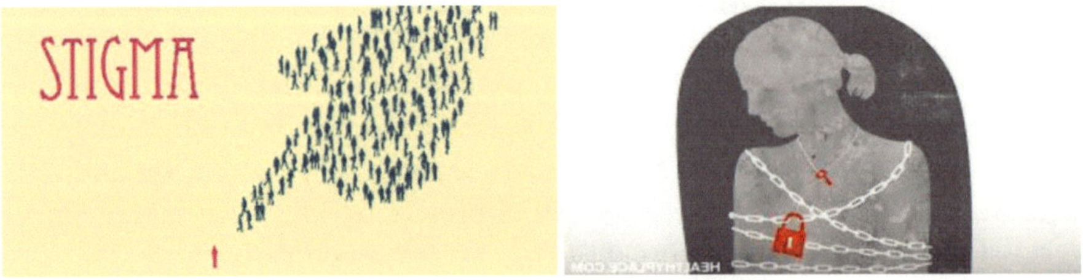

Figure 2. Social and self-stigma.

prejudiced and discriminate against them because of their mental illness or illness. It tends to stigmatize itself, create feelings of shame, and lead to worse treatment and consequence [23, 30]. If a person who suffers from depression does not feel that it is worth being treated, the people with mental illness are less likely to have proven service and treatment requirements. A research has shown that negative stereotypes, such as danger or inadequacy, are often associated with mental illness and harm people living with the illness [23]. Therefore, this can be a possible reason behind the self-stigmatization.

2.2.3. Professional stigma

Professional stigmatization refers to the fact that health care workers cause stigmatization of individual with mental disease and strengthen them. Healthcare workers do not want to be perceived as stigmatizing individual with mental illness suffering from mental illness. And for this reason, they can easily reject stigmatizing behaviors and beliefs. For this reason, it is important for professionals to become more aware of how the stigma can be predicted while working with individual with mental illnesses. Professional stigmatization may develop in a manner similar to the development of social stigmatization in the general population. Because a professional does not recognize the lack of appropriate treatment of a disabled client, he may be deprived of his rights and the individual with mental disease may become more vulnerable. This may lead them to terminate the treatment or to be treated elsewhere. Finally, professional stigmatization directed at the individual with mental disease or provider's own illness creates an obstacle to the health of the individual by preventing appropriate treatment. It may also affect the acceptance of disorders by the healthcare worker's own impersonal beliefs [24].

3. Stigma in mental health

3.1. Wrong beliefs in mental illness

Common misconceptions about mental disorders can be described as follows:

1. mental disorders, heart disease, and cancer are not real disease;
2. people who need psychiatric care should be locked away at institutions;
3. a person with a mental disorder will never be normal;
4. those with mental disorders are dangerous;
5. individuals and young people with mental disorders do not suffer;
6. those with mental disorders can work at low job levels because they are not suitable for really important or responsible positions; and
7. people with mental disorders will become ill due to their crimes [31].

3.2. Reasons for stigmatization for mental illness

The causes of stigmatization for mental illness can be individual, social, and political. Especially, it is stated that the fear factor against the individual with mental illness is the biggest factor causing the stigmatization. These individuals with mental disease are considered dangerous by society; their balance completely corrupted, when they do not know what they are going to do; they damage their environment; and they have communication problems. Another cause and one of the most important reasons is that the mental illness is not perceived as a disease. Consequently, age, gender, education, occupation, marital status, social class, culture, religious beliefs, knowledge of disease, contact with mental illness, mental illness label, type of psychopathology, characteristics of individual with mental disease, and mass media are factors affecting mental illness stigmatization [32] (**Figure 3**).

3.3. Negative consequences of stigma in mental disorders

Stigma has negative consequences for the individual in society. The stigma applied to individuals with mental disorders causes new difficulties in the individual's treatment process. Some of the symptoms of mental illness such as reluctance, lack of motivation, low motivation, and loss of self-confidence lead individuals to withdraw to their own world. While individuals try to cope with the symptoms of illness, they also have to cope with the discriminatory behavior of being stigmatized by the society. Individuals who tend to withdraw from society because of their mental illness that tends to withdraw more out of society when exposed to stigma [1].

Stigma, in mental disorders, negatively affect their confidence in themselves, their participation in the treatment, their working lives, their use of social opportunities, their ability to defend their rights in criminal justice systems, and their participation in daily life activities [33]. Concern for exposure to stigmatization leads individuals and families with mental disorders to be hesitant about treatment. This causes them not to start treatment or to leave it at the start of treatment. Failure to provide regular treatment affects the individual with mental disease recovery process badly [8]. Stigma affects many areas in the daily life of individuals. One of these is a working life. For example, employers are reluctant to recruit because they see it as aggressive, dangerous, frightening, and unreliable. At the same time, they can use insulting words in business life and question their business performance. These thoughts and behaviors prevent individuals with mental disorders from participating in the working life. Moving away from working life leads to new problems such as not being able to be in society. This situation is causing their confidence to be shaken [34].

Stigma also prevents individual with mental disorders from using as much as they can from social facilities. As well as experiencing problems in having a satisfactory job, there is also a problem with the right to live in a home on safe and appropriate conditions. In a study by Willis and colleagues, individuals with long-term mental illnesses have experienced inadequate support, living in inadequate housing conditions and showing their lives on the streets [35]. Stigma also has negative consequences within the criminal justice system. According to a study by Lamp and Weinberger [36], it has been shown that 6–15% of individuals in prison in the country have

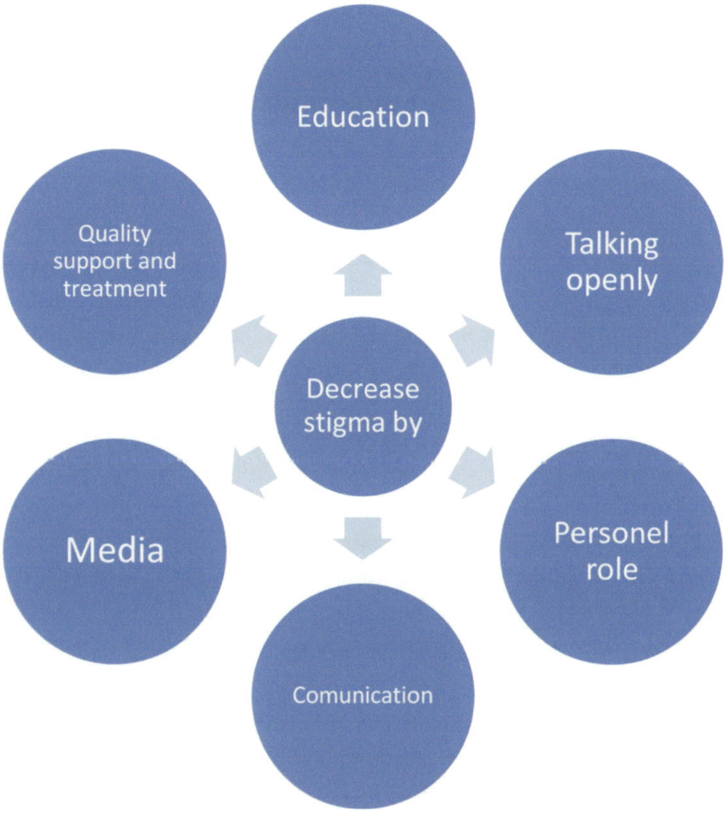

Figure 3. How to decrease stigma in society.

severe mental disorders. In a study by Watson, Corrigan, and Ottati [37] investigating the stigmatizing attitude of police officers, it has been shown that an individual with mental impairment is perceived as more dangerous. At the same time, it was revealed that the information given during the query was not reliable. While being in the criminal proceedings is difficult enough even for individuals without mental disorders, this process is more difficult for individuals and families with mental disorders and negatively affects the healing process. The stigma negatively affects the quality of life's the parents, spouses, siblings, caregivers, and people in close proximity to individuals with mental disorders. In a study by Phelan et al. [38], it was shown that families of people with mental disorders tend to conceal mental impairment from other people. Due to mental disorders in their families, they are exposed to social distance-setting behavior by the society. In summary, studies show that stigma is an obstacle for individuals with mental disorders to become active in daily life, participate in working life, and be in society.

3.4. Approaches for reducing stigma in mental diseases

1. Educational approaches to the dangers challenge false stereotypes about mental illness and change them to real knowledge. The training strategies included public service

announcements, books, flyers, films, videos, Web pages, podcasts, virtual reality, and other audiovisual support [39].

2. A second strategy for reducing stigmatization is interpersonal communication with the members of the stigmatized group. People with mental illness have the potential to reduce the prejudice levels of the general population who meet and interact with people [40].

3. Social activism or protest is the third type of stigmatization change we have examined. Protest strategies emphasize the injustices of various stigma criminals for stigmatization and discrimination: "There is protest anecdotal evidence, such as embarrassing us all to continue the idea that people with mental illness cannot look after them, are big children." Proposes that the protest can reduce harmful media representatives [41]. Psychiatry and medicine as a whole profession should develop effective methods against stigmatization of a group of mentally ill people and provide basic human rights. The relationship of psychiatry and the media, and especially the media, to psychiatry should be highly fair and professional, based on facts, not on sensation. Adequate and fair media coverage can significantly reduce the stigmatization of individual with mental disease. This can facilitate the functioning of the family and society. Therefore, changing attitudes will help people on medical care become more human and abandon negative attitudes that prevent us from becoming better and fairer [42].

4. Obsessive compulsive disorders

In OCD, we witness obsession and compulsive rituals, usually both of them. Obsessions are repetitive and ongoing thoughts impulses or beliefs which are not as simple as worries of daily life, and individual tries to ignore them through coping mechanisms as they affect daily life and cause great anxiety. People with OCD realize that all of these thoughts only exist in their minds. Permanent impulses such as unwanted thoughts or beliefs that might hurt others, getting worked up over a turned on light or an open door, and suspicions over sexual impulses can be given as examples of obsession [38, 43].

Compulsions are repetitive behaviors and mental acts, as in washing hands consecutively, repeatedly checking the task at hand, praying, and counting. For the person to have rigid rules like counting to ten is a determining factor for the behavioral aspect. Individual would feel under pressure and "compulsed" to do. Compulsions have no relation with reality; their purpose is to decrease the stress and prevent bad things from happening in the person's eye [44].

OCD leads to major difficulties in daily functioning and causes significant personality problems and mental problems when not treated. It is not surprising that the quality of life is affected by the problems encountered in functions and the nature of OCD. The social functions affecting quality of life in OCD are affected rather poorly than other mental diseases. Problems associated with intensive obsessions and compulsions affect social functions. Symptoms cause the individual to spend time with his or her family or work life. For this reason, the possibilities of positive social interaction and functional experience are reduced [45]. Anxiety may accompany obsessions and compulsions. Individuals feel themselves anxious and nervous. For this reason, the physical and social environment has an important effect on the emotional state of the individual. Both the environmental parameters and the symptoms affect each other. The anxiety that may arise from symptoms of the individual can be controlled by physical environment facilities and positive social support.

Stigma is a social force associated with people with many different health situations, feature, and social structures. Moreover, literature review shows that mental problems, sexuality, race, and STDs can also be regarded as related subjects [46]. Symptoms are not the only reason for the problems that people with psychiatric illnesses face in life. When problems these individuals live through are taken into account, stigma can be called a "second illness" [47, 48]. Individuals with psychiatric problems experience discriminatory behaviors and emotional acts in different forms. These labeling acts and situations create barriers against life opportunities for individuals. People who go through with stigmas might internalize these prejudices, in which case they start to believe that these beliefs are completely true and that creates some more barriers for them [49].

Stigma affects the people with OCD, and individuals might find themselves feeling under the weather or feel fear due to mental problem diagnosis, which can later affect the attitude toward the treatment and their motivation [47]. We see stigma as one of the many barriers we encounter on OCD treatment. Individuals with OCD go through a fear of stigma which can be described as a behavior to avoid the necessary help due to fear of a psychiatric diagnosis [50, 51] (**Figure 4**).

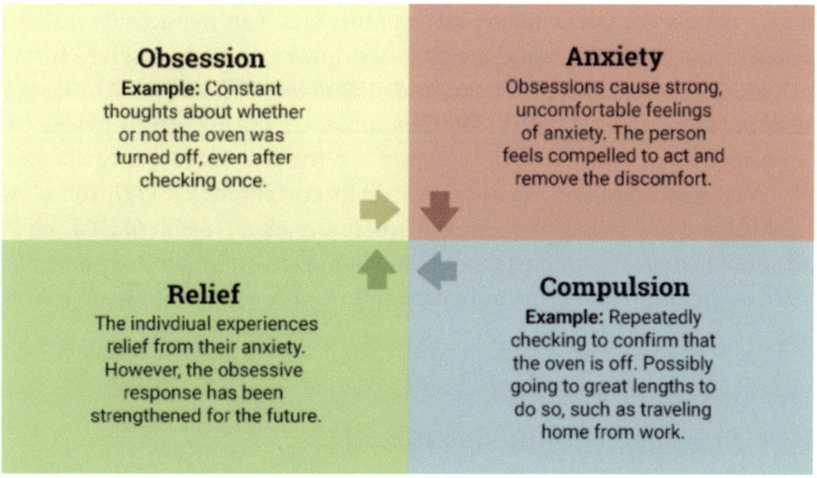

Figure 4. Obsessions and compulsions are related to anxiety and beliefs.

In society, general attitude toward people with mental issues is basically seen as "keeping away," "observation," and lastly isolation. Much of the mentioned compulsive rituals might seem unusual to the people unaware of the process individual with OCD go through. Society labels these individuals as people with strange behavior or people who act madly. The fact that labeling has started indicates that process goes to social stigma. If the person's actions are found weird but can be tolerated, they are labeled as nervous people. Stigmatized people should be evaluated according to underlying reasons behind their illnesses and their belief in themselves. Rejection of a stigmatized person depends on etiology of the illness and its interpretation [52]. CD has great significance in lives of people with OCD and their families. As the people experience increasing obsessive and compulsive thoughts, they become socially isolated, and by time, their illness gets worse and they might need to be taken care of [53, 54]. Illnesses that are treated by psychiatrists are generally regarded as mental illnesses. This term traditionally used to describe serious mental problems, and it stigmatizes people with this problem via society and themselves. Many individuals with OCD refrain from receiving necessary support because of the risk of being stigmatized. They would often look for somatic explanations such as it being a dermatological problem in order to ignore the mental problem that they have [52]. Self-stigma is a term used in the case where the individual internalizes the negative approach he/she receives. Therefore, a person with OCB who internalizes the societal prejudices would feel a flaw in themselves and therefore would expect to be rejected by the society [1, 2]. Livingston and Boyd [46] show that self-stigma affects—very strongly and negatively—the psychosocial status such as empowerment and self-esteem as much as it affects individual's psychiatric status.

Before obsessive and compulsive behaviors develop, individuals experience great trauma and intense stressful processes. Individuals' responsibilities and the value they give to events determine the significance and importance of this process. Their fear of stigma causes to hide their experiences. This situation hampers help requests, including educators and health professionals. Symptoms of OCD cause time and energy loss in the individual's life. This situation negatively affects the performance of the individuals in the activity areas that require social participation in particular. As a result, individuals isolate themselves from others [55]. Individuals with OCD often hide bullying and shame [56, 57]. They try to keep their obsessions and compulsions against future hurdles and that do not go to places that generate stress and anxiety. The presence of OCD can increase the risk of substance abuse and suicidal thoughts [58]. Attitudes and behaviors of peers are important for OCD children. As a result of negative attitudes and behaviors of peers, the possibility of exclusion of OCD children is very high. A study shows that 25% of participants are being excluded by their peers. Examples of behaviors such as kicking, hitting, rumor spreading, and social isolation are examples of peer attitudes [59].

5. Stigma in obsessive compulsive disorder

As describe above, OCD, one of mental disorders, is also adversely affected by stigma. Due to the effects of OCD, both self-attitudes and others attitudes are negatively affected stigma that can cause problems in self-esteem, seeking treatment, benefiting from social opportunities, criminal justice system, and problems in family and friends' relations. Families of individuals with OCD and close friends live difficult situations due to stigma. Self-stigma and the social stigma have a negative impact on their participation in daily life activities, their functionalities, their occupational lives, their productivity, and their social lives [33].

In individuals with OCD, emotions such as shame, guilt, and fear emerge during the first appearance of the disease. The first reaction is usually a tendency to reject. Individuals try to cope with the symptoms alone. They start to live with disease by trying to hide their symptoms. It is usually later that they perceive this as a disease. For this reason, it can be shown that they have no previous knowledge about the disease. The lack of insight causes them not seeking treatment, not getting help, and not doing research. They acknowledge that there is a trouble when it comes to coping with the symptoms, but the search for treatment with emotional factors such as shame, guilt, and fear is delayed again. OCD, like other mental disorders, is a psychiatric disorder that needs to be diagnosed and treated early. OCD diagnosis is usually delayed for such reasons. Individuals with OCD are resistant to interviewing health personnel and postpone treatment seeking. Treatment with the cause of hesitation in seeking treatment begins at a later stage of the disease. The delay in the onset of treatment affects the treatment process negatively in OCD, just as it is in other diseases. As well as having problems in seeking treatment with the cause of stigma, after the treatment starts, the treatment can also have problems with regular participation, continuity, and concluding the treatment. At the beginning of the treatment, the rate of cessation treatment in individuals is very high. Stigma slows down the process and causes them to have negative emotions. The treatment phase can be long-lasting, sometimes challenging and painful. While this process is difficult enough to cope with, the stigma makes this process even harder. **The self-perception can be changed and his belief that he is a successful cure is shaken**. The negative effect of stigmatization on patience and perseverance prevents the steady maintenance of treatment. These affect the prognosis of the disease negatively [3, 8].

Individuals with OCD experience feelings of shame, guilt, fear, and anxiety when they are diagnosed with the disease and prefer to **fight alone in the treatment process**. Fear of exposure to stigmatization prevents individuals from giving information about their illness to their relatives. In general, individuals tend to keep it confidential from the family and those close to them. This situation causes environmental support to fail. As with all other illnesses, it is important that environmental support is available to deal with the disease during the treatment process [60]. Concerns about accusations and exclusion by those who are close to the family in **relation to other people** cause problems and distances away from others [1, 61]. The tendency to keep the disease secret is caused by the inability to receive support from family members or close associates, and the prognosis of the disease is adversely affected. This is why getting help is important.

Studies show that violence and sexual obsessions are not shared in particular and that it is **more difficult to seek help** in this regard. Because of the feeling of embarrassment in these obsessions, it is delaying the search for treatment that cannot be shared with health personnel [61]. In another study, 738 adults were asked about pollution, symmetry, damage, and taboo obsessions. While symmetry obsessions were defined as OCD, subjects with taboo obsessions were exposed to stigma. Failure to have sufficient knowledge of OCD leads to the exposure of people with certain obsessions to the stigma, such as in this study [62].

Exposure to stigma, prejudiced and degrading attitudes, and discriminatory behavior of the community **negatively affect the self-esteem of individuals.** The stigma applied by the community is internalized by the individual and starts negative attitudes toward themselves. Individuals are self-stigmatizing and are beginning to label themselves. Once individuals begin to stamp themselves, they begin to diminish a sense of self-sufficiency. Later on, they do not have as much as self-confidence, self-esteem, and feeling of accomplishment, self-expression, and self-esteem. Self-esteem begins to be damaged, and the daily life of those who have problems people without self-esteem is negatively affected. Self-stigma influences their sense of success in their lives and their work life, their dissatisfaction, and their learning and development desires in the negative. They prefer to stay behind in business life, starting work, continuing, and finishing. But the problems of self-esteem and self-esteem of individuals are reducing the trust of employers. Self-stigma is also preventing participation in daily life activities. In everyday life, they are starting to refrain from carrying out activities such as communication, shopping, money management, and housekeeping. The problem that people live in self-esteem is causing their independent living skills to be negatively affected. Over time, they are becoming more dependent on their life. At the same time, they are also avoiding social activities that may be associated with other people. Their social activities such as participation in group activities, playing games, and being in contact with other people are being hurt. Self-stigma prevents the individual from making efforts on behalf of the formation of the social environment necessary to participate in social life. It leads to problems in the functionality of individuals [63, 64]. In sum, both the stigma created by other people and the stigma they apply to themselves are affecting negatively the quality of life of the individual with OCD.

Stigma also negatively affects the **relationship of individuals with their parents**. An individual may be exposed to stigma by his or her family. Having inadequate knowledge about OCD or having a false belief due to a mental illness leads the families to exclude them. They tend to reject the disease just like individuals when they first learn it. The families are starting to feel feelings such as shame, fear, anger, and guilt-like individual with OCD. This causes the individual with OCD tend to hide the signs of the disease and to hide themselves from other people. The treatment of the individual with OCD is adversely affected until the family begins to accept the disease. The fact that the parents do not see the symptoms of the disease as illness causes accusations of individuals with OCD [1, 3, 61]. During this period, the individual continues to internalize his self-labeling. The treatment of the individual is badly affected by his/her family's and self-stigma of the individual with OCD stigma thus leads to the lack of family support and the poor prognosis of the treatment.

Stigma affects **the relationship of individuals with OCD to their friends.** Individuals tend to conceal their illness from time to time, even from friends. They try to hide the symptoms of their illness by their anxiety, anger, mockery, exclusion, and stigma exposure by their friends. For this reason, they prefer to stay away from their friends in this period, to be alone. The tendency to go away, the desire to be alone, and the closure causes the individual to be left alone with this disease. In the course of treatment, environmental support is reduced in this way. At school, at home, at work, and in social life, we spend time with friends almost everywhere. Friends have an important place in everyday life. At school, at home, at work, in cinema, in theater, at the café, in sports, in social activities, etc., getting away from friends who spend time together negatively affects daily life. Exposure to stigma after sharing your illness with friends also affects individual with OCD's life negatively. The lack of knowledge and misunderstandings about OCD causes the symptoms of the illness to be perceived by the individual as deliberate behavior, and the individual's friends may expose them to stigma in this case. It adversely affects the ability of the individual to perform daily life activities, productivity, occupational performance, and leisure activities. This causes the individual's self-esteem to be impaired and the prognosis of the treatment to deteriorate [3, 62]. Persons who are friends with individuals with OCD are also exposed to stigma. People tend to think that they have the same behavior as individuals whose OCD is their friends. The personal characteristics and wrong evaluations attributed to the stamped individual are also attributed to the friends of these individuals. This situation also causes bad influence on friendship relations. The stigmatized individual's friends lead him away from him, leaving him alone and weakening the friendship relationship. The daily lives, productions, social activities, and social support of the stamped individuals are negatively affected on the treatment process [3, 62].

OCD is a psychological disorder that **affects daily life for individuals and their families**. The general attitude of society to this disease is to stay away at first. Individuals with OCD start struggle in their daily lives because of indecisiveness, self-reliance, and disruptive behaviors. As individuals with OCD become more difficult to manage their daily lives, the individual with OCD' families are starting to do it on their behalf. But sometimes families also begin not to deal with the tasks and activities of individual with OCD. For this reason, families feel stressed to take more responsibility for the daily life activities of the OCD individual [1]. Family members of individuals with mental disability are also exposed to stigmatization. Negative personal characteristics directed to the individual with OCD are also mirrored to the relatives of the individual with OCD. Families are shown as defective, guilty, and embarrassed. Recently, studies have been carried out on the stigma that the family is exposed to. Surveys reveal that they are worthless and humiliated because they are family members of the person with a mental disorder. The families exposed to stigma are under the pressure of the society. This increases the stress and anxiety of the family. Stress, anxiety, social stigma, can also cause mental ill effects on the family. Family stigmatization leads to a negative impact on both the relationship between the individual with OCD and the family as well as the relationship with society. They are moving away from society, starting to be alone and living in environmental constraints. Because of family stigma, family members are getting away from school, work, and outside, and their social participation is decreased [1, 65, 66].

The treatment process can be a lengthy and challenging process. It may become a situation that consumes the family and the individual with OCD. In the meantime, the family and the individual with OCD should be supported mentally well. Stigma can prevent with this support from family and individual with OCD. Negative attitudes toward the family influence the individual, giving the right support in the treatment process. Moreover, they are influenced negatively psychologically and socially. The inability of the family members to support as much as their ability to handle leads to slowing and prolonging the prognosis. At the same time, some of the destructive effects of the disease increase, causing negative attitudes about the process [1, 65, 66]. In summary, stigma on family of person with OCD; adversely affects family, person with OCD and their relationship.

5.1. Negative consequences of stigma in children with obsessive compulsive disorder

Stigma not only affects adults but also youth and children. Since the incidence of OCD is lower in children, there is not much research done on them. Obsessions and compulsions seen in children affect their daily routines, family relationships, friendship relationships, and self-esteem. The self-esteem of children exposed to stigma by their friends is negatively affected. This causes many problems to emerge, in children, as in adults. Reduced self-esteem caused experiencing problems such as having trouble with going to school, not doing homework, not having friendship relationship, closing up, and difficulty to participate in the treatment.

Stigma also negatively affects children's friendship relationship. The play takes an important place in the child's life. Friends are needed to play games. Exposure to stigma among friends is causing them to move away. The game environment of a child who is away from friends is disappearing. Moreover, friendship relationship improves the level of stress of the child and loneliness. The exposure of the child to stigma causes nervous, angry, and anxious behaviors. The family of the child, whose stress level is increasing, is also negatively affected by this situation [67, 68].

The family that is exposed to the child's stigma is also exposed to stigmatization. Family stigma causes family relations to be influenced, family members to be affected by the friendship relationship, and the level of family stress to be increased. The fact that the parents try to cope with these stress factors negatively affect their participation in the long treatment process of the child. Such problems caused by stigma are adversely affecting the treatment process in children, as well as in adults. Because of stigma, diminished supportive mechanisms, increased stress, emotional impact of the child, and problem of participation in the game are problematic in the progress of the treatment process [69].

6. Psychosocial interventions for stigma

In OCD management, medical perspective is dominant in general sense [70, 71]. However, OCD people continue their lives in society beyond medical drug treatment. Stigma is often referred to as secondary disease [48]. For this reason, it is important to have a biopsychosocial approach to OCD. Occupational therapists use the biopsychosocial and holistic approach for clients. In the following sections, individuals with OCD are referred to as *client*. For occupational therapy, it is important that the clients fulfill his roles, participation in occupations, and social participation and existence as an individual [72]. Occupational therapists do individual and/or community-based interventions to combat self-stigma, professional stigma, and social stigma that individuals are exposed to. Interventions to be conducted to client centered can be classified as promotion self-awareness, coping strategies, and encouragement. Interventions for social and professional stigma can be classified as occupational justice, community-based rehabilitation, education, and support groups.

"Self-stigma interventions can be classified promotion self-awareness, coping strategies and encouragement."

6.1. Promotion self-awareness

In mental illness, individuals may not be aware of self-stigmatization. Because of wrong beliefs or thoughts about themselves, they may have difficulty in performing their roles and participating in their daily activities. For this reason, it is important to increase insight and to create individual awareness in reducing stigmatization. Occupational therapists can use cognitive behavioral therapy, psychoeducation, and also photovoice methods to help clients write and express their thoughts and behaviors who have difficulty in verbally expressing in order to provide individual awareness; thus, contributing to the client's occupational identity and avoiding self-stigmatization.

Cognitive behavioral therapy involves changing individuals' misconceptions with the right thinking. In this regard, it is accepted as a direct and permanent method. CBT, which is used in combination with medical treatment in many mental disorders, is highly effective. CBT, the most commonly used method of treating person with OCD, also has a significant role in reducing self-stigmatization [73, 74]. This method, which is widely used in OCD seen in children, helps to prevent the self-stigma that the individual applies to himself [75, 76]. CBT can be done individually or in groups [77]. Reaching of cognitive behavioral treatment is difficult because of the lack of specialized therapists in the field of reaching. Occupational therapists can specialize in this area to help OCD individuals overcome self-regulation. In addition, CBT is cost effective and accessible via the Internet [78].

One of the most important causes of self-stigmatization is having missing or incorrect information about the disease. Also, diagnosis can lead to labeling in individuals. Psychoeducation is one of the most effective and widely used method as CBT. Even brief information reduces the violence and social distance applied to the individual with OCD. The aim of this pyschoeducation is to give information about the individual's illnesses, to reduce the self-labeling, and to raise the inner awareness of the client. In the context of ideal psychoeducation; medical, psychological, and sociological information about the disease should be included, information about treatment and process should be given, strategies for coping should be explained, and practical training should be done. In addition to these contexts, stories of individuals on similar conditions may increase the effectiveness of education. Occupational therapists can provide these trainings in community mental health centers, hospitals, OCD associations, or individuals with OCD who consultate to them [79].

Photovoice methods used for clients are actively involved in reflecting their lives through photography/draw picture and group work. Photovoice methods enable the individual to increase his/her inner awareness and understand the conditions of the disease and the obstacle [80]. Very few studies have focused on photovoice methods to prevent stigmatization and participatory approaches [81]. Nonetheless, the photovoice methods can be used to understand the paradoxical relationship between social stigma and ethical values. Kawa model developed by Iwama is a photovoice occupational therapy model. This model enables the individual to demonstrate a direct relationship with culture [82]. The client describes the situations in which the individual perceives their own life as difficulty or opportunity in his Kawa drawings. For this reason, in occupational therapy, Kawa River model can be used as an evaluation and intervention in providing stigma awareness. Bavaro has used the Model of Human Occupation [MOHO] to deeply understand the client with OCD. He stated that habits, rituals, environment, and an occupational therapy model can be used for evaluation and intervention of an individual's occupational identity and performance [83]. With the MOHO model, occupational therapist can help to client to reconstruct his own occupational identity and find the source of inner motivation.

Also, Garland noted that in his study, animal-assisted therapy promotes family and individual communication, contributes to participation, and reduces stigmatization of the disease due to this signification and normalization [84]. Occupational therapist can use purposeful occupations such as animal-assisted approaches to increase social participation of the client and to facilitate social relationships.

6.2. Coping strategies

Obsessions and compulsions and related maladaptive behaviors are the most common causes for individuals to social and self-stigma. Management of obsessions and compulsions are thought to diminish the problems encountered in social participation. Occupational therapists play a pivotal role in teaching different coping strategies and in providing effective use of these coping strategies in different environments and conditions with motor learning principles. Coping strategies can be classified relaxation techniques, body awareness, time management, and desensitization.

Relaxation techniques, which have 35.9% of the strategies used in OCD individuals, are frequently used in the management of anxiety disorders resulting in obsessions and compulsions [85, 86]. Relaxation techniques have been reported to cause somatic and cognitive components to relapse in obsessive compulsive disorders [87]. However, there is still a need for more study for OCD. Relaxation techniques control the repetitive rituals of individuals in their participation and therefore suggest that they can be protected from stigma. Occupational therapist specializing in body–mind awareness and relaxation techniques is needed. By promoting mind and body integration with the biopsychosocial approach, increase in body awareness is thought to have a positive effect on clients' own thoughts.

Time is an important concept in the management of obsessions and compulsions seen in OCD. Participation of daily activities or social activities needs requirements for performance patterns. In occupational therapy, performance patterns define roles, habits, and routines. Beyond these performance patterns, there is also requirement for time management. Occupational therapists conduct an activity analysis to reveal the personal, environmental, and activity demands that activities require. The division of activities into tasks, followed by these steps, allows the regulation of the rituals of clients with OCD. However, occupational therapists teach OCD individuals time management techniques.

Sensory processing disorders in childhood may lead to excessive ritual behaviors. Children with tactile hypersensitivity were found to have an OC tendency later in life, and oral and tactile hypersensitivity in adults were associated with obsessions and compulsions. Studies of OCD on sensory processing both in childhood and on adult individuals show that desensitization techniques are effective on obsessions and compulsions [88–90]. In occupational therapy, sensory integration therapy and desensitization techniques in children and adults and the environment they live in have an important role in enabling individuals to cope with symptoms, fulfill their roles, and interact with the environment. These methods are thought to reduce stigmatization.

Individuals with OCD are also stigmatizing in their treatment seeking or avoiding treatment seeking because they are stigmatizing [91, 92]. Within this paradox, clients' attainment of treatment and social inclusion are affected [30]. Occupational therapists should encourage individuals to participate in activities and manage health [72]. Encouraging clients with OCD is an important intervention to remove the negative consequences of the stigma.

For social and professional stigma, occupational therapy interventions can be categorized as providing occupational justice, community-based rehabilitation, education and support groups.

The concept of occupational justice argues that individuals have activity capacities, needs, and routines in their environments and have the right to use these capacities to maintain their lives and social participation and empowerment social inclusion [93, 94]. Stigma inhibits social inclusion in OCD individuals [47]. In occupational justice framework; occupational balance and occupational deprivation terms have been used. Occupational deprivation refers to the deprivation of the purposeful occupations the clients is doing due to social factors over time; the occupational alienation refers to estrangement, loss control, and sense of isolation due to social or self-conditions, while the clients fulfill their occupations and roles, and the occupational imbalance, in which there is an imbalance between the occupations required by the roles and the time allocated. Occupational deprivation and occupational alienation are inevitable for OCD due to stigma. The stigma in OCD needs to be considered in the context of occupational science.

Community-based psychiatric rehabilitation aims to provide rehabilitation services and sustainable services within the society and culture in which the individual lives. Studies about people with OCD and society can be effective in changing the cultural history of stigmatization. Projects supported by volunteers can also influence the cultural sub-structure of the stigma [95]. Occupational therapists can conduct community-based rehabilitation work and contribute to the social consensus of clients [96]. Community-based rehabilitation practice with an occupational justice conception that will provide social participation and reduce stigma is among the interventions occupational therapists will have [97]. Community participation, social inclusion, and occupational engagement are highly important occupational therapy interventions for reducing stigma and discrimination [98].

Occupational therapists visit the home where the client lives and make the home assessments. OT can provide OCD management and can make appropriate house arrangements for the client. The family and/or caregiver are informed. For school-aged OCD clients, OTs can visit the school, be informed by interviewing their peers and their teachers and if necessary, make appropriate environmental adjustments to the client. Informing adults and making workplace visits and environmental adaptations for clients with OCD have an important place in interventions that can reduce stigmatization.

Anti-stigma or reducing stigmatization interventions focused on the people with OCD and their families, health professionals, the general public, pupils and teachers, and health professionals. Education about OCD and misbeliefs is the primary aim of most campaigns, followed by the empowerment of people OCD and the prevention of impact of stigmatization [99, 100]. Occupational therapists have an advocacy role to promote social awareness and support the social integration of clients [72]. For OCD, occupational therapists can make these campaigns at a social level, and they can argue with politicians for legal regulations. It is among the responsibilities of occupational therapists to defend the rights of clients and to ensure the participation of clients with OCD in this way.

The media, however, play an important role in determining the attitudes of individuals toward perceptions and stigma and have a growing voice [101]. TV programs and publications have been reported to have positive effects on stigma [102]. A study on media reported that the Monk character, an individual with OCD, reduced stigma against OCD [60]. In the technology world, there are many people who reach through social media and individuals can be encouraged to tell their stories by digital storytelling methods. Thus, stigmatization can be decreased by increasing social awareness [103].

It has been noted that individuals with OCD have avoided treatment seeking because of the stigma they have seen most from their families. More stigma is reported to be applied especially in socio-demographic lower income families [104]. Also, family members living with the patient (such as parents, partners, children and siblings) are involved in daily rituals and undergoing social stigmatization. For this reason, families may encounter inequalities in occupational role performing. It is possible for OCD individuals to have access to treatment and to support their social integration and to provide social inclusion for the OCD individual's family members. The biggest profit from the support groups could have individuals with high levels of self-stigmatization and poor social networks. Such groups might be focused on stigmatization (and thus indirectly on building self-esteem). The biggest profits from the support groups were the high levels of self-stigmatization and poor social networks. Educational activities are of great importance as such groups might be focused on stigmatization (and thus indirectly on building self-esteem), adaptive coping strategies to deal with daily hassles and interpersonal conflicts, and adopting supportive behaviors. These trainings can be made for health professionals for professional stigma, for children and adolescents with OCD [105], or for general public [100].

Taking social support from family and peers is the way to reduce the social stigma that families are going through. In many countries, support groups have been established for OCD individuals and their families. Bringing together individuals who live in similar conditions allows a group to become less isolated from society [106]. Children learn from their peers. Child or adolescent peer groups are also important in the context of the participation of children [80]. Web-based systems can communicate with social media [103] or virtual-based systems can be effective. The direction of occupational therapists to social support groups and peer support groups is the occupational therapy interventions that promote social integration of clients and thus reduce stigma [79, 106].

The best approach to reduce stigma should be a holistic approach and community-based rehabilitation to control clients' symptoms, to protect the clients' occupational identity, to tackle the client and the living environment together, and to raise the awareness of the clients, family, and the community.

Author details

Gokcen Akyurek*, Kubra Sahadet Sezer, Leyla Kaya and Kezban Temucin

*Address all correspondence to: gkcnakyrk@gmail.com

Department of Occupational Therapy, Faculty of Health Science, Hacettepe University, Ankara, Turkey

References

[1] Ociskova M, Prasko J, Sedlackova Z. Stigma and self-stigma in patients with anxiety disorders. Activitas Nervosa Superior Rediviva. 2013;**55**(1-2):12-18

[2] Corrigan PW, Rowan D, Green A, Lundin R, River P, Uphoff-Wasowski K, et al. Challenging two mental illness stigmas: Personal responsibility and dangerousness. Schizophrenia Bulletin. 2002;**28**(2):293-309

[3] Corrigan P. How stigma interferes with mental health care. The American Psychologist. 2004;**59**(7):614

[4] Anthony WA, Blanch A. Supported employment for persons who are psychiatrically disabled: An historical and conceptual perspective. Psychosocial Rehabilitation Journal. 1987;**11**(2):5

[5] Sturm R, Gresenz CR, Pacula RL, Wells KB. Datapoints: Labor force participation by persons with mental illness. Psychiatric Services. 1999;**50**(11):1407

[6] Corrigan PW. Target-specific stigma change: A strategy for impacting mental illness stigma. Psychiatric Rehabilitation Journal. 2004;**28**(2):113

[7] Holmes EP, River LP. Individual strategies for coping with the stigma of severe mental illness. Cognitive and Behavioral Practice. 1998;**5**(2):231-239

[8] Hayward P, Bright JA. Stigma and mental illness: A review and critique. Journal of Mental Health. 1997

[9] Vogel DL, Wade NG, Haake S. Measuring the self-stigma associated with seeking psychological help. Journal of Counseling Psychology. 2006;**53**(3):325

[10] Vogel DL, Wade NG, Ascheman PL. Measuring perceptions of stigmatization by others for seeking psychological help: Reliability and validity of a new stigma scale with college students. Journal of Counseling Psychology. 2009;**56**(2):301

[11] Chang KH, Horrocks S. Lived experiences of family caregivers of mentally ill relatives. Journal of Advanced Nursing. 2006;**53**(4):435-443

[12] Steele A, Maruyama N, Galynker I. Psychiatric symptoms in caregivers of patients with bipolar disorder: A review. Journal of Affective Disorders. 2010;**121**(1-2):10-21

[13] Markarian Y, Larson MJ, Aldea MA, Baldwin SA, Good D, Berkeljon A, et al. Multiple pathways to functional impairment in obsessive–compulsive disorder. Clinical Psychology Review. 2010;**30**(1):78-88

[14] Bobes J, Gonzalez M, Bascaran M, Arango C, Saiz P, Bousono M. Quality of life and disability in patients with obsessive-compulsive disorder. European Psychiatry. 2001; **16**(4):239-245

[15] LeBel TP. Perceptions of and responses to stigma. Sociology Compass. 2008;**2**(2):409-432

[16] Sayers J. The world health report 2001-mental health: New understanding, new hope. Bulletin of the World Health Organization. 2001;**79**:1085

[17] Şemin S, Aras Ş. Temel yönleriyle psikiyatride etik: Dokuz eylül yayınları; 2004

[18] Taşkin EO. Damgalama, ayrimcilik ve ruhsal hastalik. Psikiyatri Psikoloji Psikofarmakoloji Dergisi; 2004

[19] Goffman E. Stigma: Notes on the Management of Spoiled Identity. Simon and Schuster; 2009

[20] Goffman E. Stigma: The Management of Spoiled Identities. New York: Simon and Schuster; 1963

[21] Gary FA. Stigma: Barrier to mental health care among ethnic minorities. Issues in Mental Health Nursing. 2005;**26**(10):979-999

[22] Bulanda JJ, Bruhn C, Byro-Johnson T, Zentmyer M. Addressing mental health stigma among young adolescents: Evaluation of a youth-led approach. Health and Social Work. 2014;**39**(2):73-80

[23] Corrigan PW, Morris SB, Michaels PJ, Rafacz JD, Rüsch N. Challenging the public stigma of mental illness: A meta-analysis of outcome studies. Psychiatric Services. 2012; **63**(10):963-973

[24] Ahmedani BK. Mental health stigma: Society, individuals, and the profession. Journal of Social Work Values and Ethics. 2011;**8**(2):4-1

[25] Bishop TF, Seirup JK, Pincus HA, Ross JS. Population of US practicing psychiatrists declined, 2003-13, which may help explain poor access to mental health care. Health Affairs. 2016;**35**(7):1271-1277

[26] Holt R, Peveler R. Diabetes and cardiovascular risk in severe mental illness: A missed opportunity and challenge for the future. Practical Diabetes International. 2010; **27**(2):79-84ii

[27] Wallace A. Public Attitudes to Housing. Joseph Rowntree Foundation York; 2010

[28] Yang LH, Kleinman A, Link BG, Phelan JC, Lee S, Good B. Culture and stigma: Adding moral experience to stigma theory. Social Science and Medicine. 2007;**64**(7):1524-1535

[29] Cheon BK, Chiao JY. Cultural variation in implicit mental illness stigma. Journal of Cross-Cultural Psychology. 2012;**43**(7):1058-1062

[30] Clement S, Schauman O, Graham T, Maggioni F, Evans-Lacko S, Bezborodovs N, et al. What is the impact of mental health-related stigma on help-seeking? A systematic review of quantitative and qualitative studies. Psychological Medicine. 2015;**45**(1):11-27

[31] Schulze B, Angermeyer MC. Subjective experiences of stigma. A focus group study of schizophrenic patients, their relatives and mental health professionals. Social Science and Medicine. 2003;**56**(2):299-312

[32] Çam O, Çuhadar D. Ruhsal hastalığa sahip bireylerde damgalama süreci ve içselleştirilmiş damgalama. Psikiyatri Hemşireliği Dergisi. 2011;**2**(3):136-140

[33] Sickel AE, Seacat JD, Nabors NA. Mental health stigma update: A review of consequences. Advances in Mental Health. 2014;**12**(3):202-215

[34] Brohan E, Henderson C, Little K, Thornicroft G. Employees with mental health problems: Survey of UK employers' knowledge, attitudes and workplace practices. Epidemiology and Psychiatric Sciences. 2010;**19**(4):326-332

[35] Willis AG, Willis GB, Male A, Henderson M, Manderscheid R. Mental Illness and Disability in the US Adult Household Population. Mental Health, United States1998. pp. 235-246

[36] Lamb HR, Weinberger LE. Persons with severe mental illness in jails and prisons: A review. Psychiatric Services. 1998;**49**(4):483-492

[37] Watson AC, Corrigan PW, Ottati V. Police officers' attitudes toward and decisions about persons with mental illness. Psychiatric Services. 2004;**55**(1):49-53

[38] Phelan JC, Bromet EJ, Link BG. Psychiatric illness and family stigma. Schizophrenia Bulletin. 1998;**24**(1):115-126

[39] Finkelstein J, Lapshin O, Wasserman E. Randomized study of different anti-stigma media. Patient Education and Counseling. 2008;**71**(2):204-214

[40] Corrigan PW. On the Stigma of Mental Illness: Practical Strategies for Research and Social Change. American Psychological Association; 2005

[41] Wahl OF. Media Madness: Public Images of Mental Illness. Rutgers University Press; 1997

[42] Babic D. Stigma and mental illness. Materia Socio-Medica. 2010;**22**(1):43

[43] Abramowitz JS, Taylor S, McKay D. Obsessive-compulsive disorder. The Lancet. 2009; **374**(9688):491-499

[44] Association AP. Diagnostic and Statistical Manual of Mental Disorders (DSM-5®). American Psychiatric Pub; 2013

[45] Kugler BB, Lewin AB, Phares V, Geffken GR, Murphy TK, Storch EA. Quality of life in obsessive-compulsive disorder: The role of mediating variables. Psychiatry Research. 2013;**206**(1):43-49

[46] Livingston JD, Boyd JE. Correlates and consequences of internalized stigma for people living with mental illness: A systematic review and meta-analysis. Social Science and Medicine. 2010;**71**(12):2150-2161

[47] Ociskova M, Prasko J, Cerna M, Jelenova D, Kamaradova D, Latalova K, et al. Obsessive compulsive disorder and stigmatization. Activitas Nervosa Superior Rediviva. 2013; **55**(1-2):19-26

[48] Finzen A. "Der Verwaltungsrat ist schizophren": Die Krankheit und das Stigma. Psychiatrie-Verlag; 1996

[49] Abramowitz JS. Understanding and Treating Obsessive-Compulsive Disorder: A Cognitive Behavioral Approach. Routledge; 2006

[50] García-Soriano G, Rufer M, Delsignore A, Weidt S. Factors associated with non-treatment or delayed treatment seeking in OCD sufferers: A review of the literature. Psychiatry Research. 2014;**220**(1-2):1-10

[51] Rüsch N, Angermeyer MC, Corrigan PW. Mental illness stigma: Concepts, consequences, and initiatives to reduce stigma. European Psychiatry. 2005;**20**(8):529-539

[52] Praško J, Mainerová B, Diveky T, Kamarádová D, Jelenová D, Grambal A, et al. Panic disorder and stigmatization. Activitas Nervosa Superior Rediviva. 2011;**53**(4):194-201

[53] Barrett P, Healy-Farrell L, March JS. Cognitive-behavioral family treatment of childhood obsessive-compulsive disorder: A controlled trial. Journal of the American Academy of Child and Adolescent Psychiatry. 2004;**43**(1):46-62

[54] Stengler-Wenzke K, Trosbach J, Dietrich S, Angermeyer MC. Coping strategies used by the relatives of people with obsessive–compulsive disorder. Journal of Advanced Nursing. 2004;**48**(1):35-42

[55] Keyes C, Nolte L, Williams TI. The battle of living with obsessive compulsive disorder: A qualitative study of young people's experiences. Child and Adolescent Mental Health. 2017

[56] Helbing M-LC, Ficca M. Obsessive-compulsive disorder in school-age children. The Journal of School Nursing. 2009;**25**(1):15-26

[57] Leininger M, Taylor Dyches T, Prater MA, Heath MA. Teaching students with obsessive-compulsive disorder. Intervention in School and Clinic. 2010;**45**(4):221-231

[58] Sloman GM, Gallant J, Storch EA. A school-based treatment model for pediatric obsessive-compulsive disorder. Child Psychiatry and Human Development. 2007;**38**(4):303-319

[59] Chaturvedi A, Murdick NL, Gartin BC. Obsessive compulsive disorder: What an educator needs to know. Physical Disabilities: Education and Related Services. 2014;**33**(2):71-83

[60] Fennell D, Boyd M. Obsessive-compulsive disorder in the media. Deviant Behavior. 2014;**35**(9):669-686

[61] Glazier K, Wetterneck C, Singh S, Williams M. Stigma and shame as barriers to treatment for obsessive-compulsive and related disorders. Journal of Depression and Anxiety. 2015;**4**(191):2167. DOI: 1044.1000191

[62] McCarty RJ, Guzick AG, Swan LK, McNamara JP. Stigma and recognition of different types of symptoms in OCD. Journal of Obsessive-Compulsive and Related Disorders. 2017;**12**:64-70

[63] Corrigan PW, Watson AC, Barr L. The self–stigma of mental illness: Implications for self-esteem and self-efficacy. Journal of Social and Clinical Psychology. 2006;**25**(8):875-884

[64] Link BG, Phelan JC. Conceptualizing stigma. Annual Review of Sociology. 2001;**27**(1): 363-385

[65] Corrigan PW, Miller FE. Shame, blame, and contamination: A review of the impact of mental illness stigma on family members. Journal of Mental Health. 2004;**13**(6):537-548

[66] Corrigan PW, Watson AC, Miller FE. Blame, shame, and contamination: The impact of mental illness and drug dependence stigma on family members. Journal of Family Psychology. 2006;**20**(2):239

[67] Piacentini J, Langley AK. Cognitive-behavioral therapy for children who have obsessive-compulsive disorder. Journal of Clinical Psychology. 2004;**60**(11):1181-1194

[68] Futh A, Simonds LM, Micali N. Obsessive-compulsive disorder in children and adolescents: Parental understanding, accommodation, coping and distress. Journal of Anxiety Disorders. 2012;**26**(5):624-632

[69] Abedi MR, Vostanis P. Evaluation of quality of life therapy for parents of children with obsessive–compulsive disorders in Iran. European Child and Adolescent Psychiatry. 2010;**19**(7):605-613

[70] Baldwin DS, Anderson IM, Nutt DJ, Allgulander C, Bandelow B, den Boer JA, et al. Evidence-based pharmacological treatment of anxiety disorders, post-traumatic stress disorder and obsessive-compulsive disorder: A revision of the 2005 guidelines from the British Association for Psychopharmacology. Journal of Psychopharmacology. 2014;**28**(5):403-439

[71] Bandelow B, Zohar J, Hollander E, Kasper S, Möller H-J, Disorders WTFoTGfAO-CP-TS, et al. World Federation of Societies of biological psychiatry (WFSBP) guidelines for the pharmacological treatment of anxiety, obsessive-compulsive and post-traumatic stress disorders–first revision. The World Journal of Biological Psychiatry. 2008;**9**(4):248-312

[72] Amini DA, Kannenberg K, Bodison S, Chang P, Colaianni D, Goodrich B, et al. Occupational therapy practice framework: Domain & process 3rd edition. The American Journal of Occupational Therapy. 2014;**68**:S1-S48

[73] Hofmann SG, Asnaani A, Vonk IJ, Sawyer AT, Fang A. The efficacy of cognitive behavioral therapy: A review of meta-analyses. Cognitive Therapy and Research. 2012;**36**(5):427-440

[74] McKay D, Sookman D, Neziroglu F, Wilhelm S, Stein DJ, Kyrios M, et al. Efficacy of cognitive-behavioral therapy for obsessive–compulsive disorder. Psychiatry Research. 2015;**225**(3):236-246

[75] Babinski DE, Pelham WE Jr, Waxmonsky JG. Cognitive-behavioral therapy for pediatric obsessive-compulsive disorder complicated by stigma: A case study. Clinical Case Studies. 2014;**13**(1):95-110

[76] March JS, Mulle K. OCD in Children and Adolescents: A Cognitive-Behavioral Treatment Manual. Guilford Press; 1998

[77] Yanos PT, Roe D, Lysaker PH. Narrative enhancement and cognitive therapy: A new group-based treatment for internalized stigma among persons with severe mental illness. International Journal of Group Psychotherapy. 2011;**61**(4):576-595

[78] Patel SR, Wheaton MG, Andersson E, Rück C, Schmidt AB, La Lima CN, et al. Acceptability, feasibility, and effectiveness of internet-based cognitive-behavioral therapy for obsessive-compulsive disorder in New York. Behavior Therapy;**2017**

[79] Piacentini J, Bergman RL, Chang S, Langley A, Peris T, Wood JJ, et al. Controlled comparison of family cognitive behavioral therapy and psychoeducation/relaxation training for child obsessive-compulsive disorder. Journal of the American Academy of Child and Adolescent Psychiatry. 2011;**50**(11):1149-1161

[80] Russinova Z, Rogers ES, Gagne C, Bloch P, Drake KM, Mueser KT. A randomized controlled trial of a peer-run antistigma photovoice intervention. Psychiatric Services. 2014;**65**(2):242-246

[81] Lal S, Jarus T, Suto MJ. A scoping review of the photovoice method: Implications for occupational therapy research. Canadian Journal of Occupational Therapy. 2012;**79**(3):181-190

[82] Iwama MK. The Kawa (River) Model: Client Centred Rehabilitation in Cultural Context. Rehabilitation. Elsevier; 2006. pp. 147-168

[83] Bavaro SM. Occupational therapy and obsessive-compulsive disorder. The American Journal of Occupational Therapy. 1991;**45**(5):456-458

[84] Garland C, Hayik S, Machonis C, McDonough C, Johnson C. Emotional Effects of Pet Facilitated Therapy on Hospice Residents. College Misericordia: Unpublished masters project Dallas; 1997

[85] Jacobson NC, Newman MG, Goldfried MR. Clinical feedback about empirically supported treatments for obsessive-compulsive disorder. Behavior Therapy. 2016;**47**(1):75-90

[86] Gava I, Barbui C, Aguglia E, Carlino D, Churchill R, De Vanna M, et al. Psychological treatments versus treatment as usual for obsessive compulsive disorder (OCD). Cochrane Database of Systematic Reviews. 2007;**2**

[87] Sarris J, Camfield D, Berk M. Complementary medicine, self-help, and lifestyle interventions for obsessive compulsive disorder (OCD) and the OCD spectrum: A systematic review. Journal of Affective Disorders. 2012;**138**(3):213-221

[88] Dar R, Kahn DT, Carmeli R. The relationship between sensory processing, childhood rituals and obsessive–compulsive symptoms. Journal of Behavior Therapy and Experimental Psychiatry. 2012;**43**(1):679-684

[89] Rieke EF, Anderson D. Adolescent/adult sensory profile and obsessive-compulsive disorder. The American Journal of Occupational Therapy. 2009;**63**(2):138

[90] Whittal ML, Woody SR, McLean PD, Rachman S, Robichaud M. Treatment of obsessions: A randomized controlled trial. Behaviour Research and Therapy. 2010;**48**(4):295-303

[91] Belloch A, del Valle G, Morillo C, Carrió C, Cabedo E. To seek advice or not to seek advice about the problem: The help-seeking dilemma for obsessive-compulsive disorder. Social Psychiatry and Psychiatric Epidemiology. 2009;**44**(4):257

[92] Overton SL, Medina SL. The stigma of mental illness. Journal of Counseling and Development. 2008;**86**(2):143-151

[93] Stadnyk R. Occupational Justice. An Introduction to Occupation. The Art and Science of Living; 2010. pp. 329-358

[94] Nilsson I, Townsend E. Occupational justice—Bridging theory and practice. Scandinavian Journal of Occupational Therapy. 2010;**17**(1):57-63

[95] Heijnders M, Van, Der Meij S. The fight against stigma: An overview of stigma-reduction strategies and interventions. Psychology Health and Medicine. 2006;**11**(3):353-363

[96] Scaffa ME, Reitz SM. Occupational Therapy Community-Based Practice Settings. FA Davis; 2013

[97] Durocher E, Gibson BE, Rappolt S. Occupational justice: A conceptual review. Journal of Occupational Science. 2014;**21**(4):418-430

[98] McKay E, Craik C, Lim KH, Richards G. Advancing Occupational Therapy in Mental Health Practice. John Wiley & Sons; 2014

[99] Beldie A, Den Boer JA, Brain C, Constant E, Figueira ML, Filipcic I, et al. Fighting stigma of mental illness in midsize European countries. Social Psychiatry and Psychiatric Epidemiology. 2012;**47**(1):1-38

[100] Warman DM, Phalen PL, Martin JM. Impact of a brief education about mental illness on stigma of OCD and violent thoughts. Journal of Obsessive-Compulsive and Related Disorders. 2015;**5**:16-23

[101] Gherman A, Predescu E, Iftene F, Cadariu AA. The role of media in anti-stigma campaigns. Anti-stigma campaign: A brief research report for obsessive compulsive disorder and specific phobia. Journal of Cognitive and Behavioral Psychotherapies. 2008;**8**(2)

[102] Davidson T, Moreland A, Bunnell BE, Winkelmann J, Hamblen JL, Ruggiero KJ. Reducing Stigma in Mental Health through Digital Storytelling. Deconstructing Stigma in Mental Health. IGI Global; 2018. pp. 169-183

[103] Betton V, Borschmann R, Docherty M, Coleman S, Brown M, Henderson C. The role of social media in reducing stigma and discrimination. The British Journal of Psychiatry. 2015;**206**(6):443-444

[104] Geffken GR, Storch EA, Duke DC, Monaco L, Lewin AB, Goodman WK. Hope and coping in family members of patients with obsessive-compulsive disorder. Journal of Anxiety Disorders. 2006;**20**(5):614-629

[105] Pinfold V, Toulmin H, Thornicroft G, Huxley P, Farmer P, Graham T. Reducing psychiatric stigma and discrimination: Evaluation of educational interventions in UK secondary schools. The British Journal of Psychiatry. 2003;**182**(4):342-346

[106] Söchting I, Third B. Behavioral group treatment for obsessive-compulsive disorder in adolescence: A pilot study. International Journal of Group Psychotherapy. 2011; **61**(1):84-97

Section 5

Therapy Modalities of Anxiety Disorders

Chapter 7

Cognitive Behavior Therapy and Mindfulness-Based Intervention for Social Anxiety Disorder

Kentaro Shirotsuki and Shota Noda

Additional information is available at the end of the chapter

http://dx.doi.org/10.5772/intechopen.79345

Abstract

Social anxiety disorder (SAD) is a marked, or intense, fear or anxiety of social situations in which the individual may be scrutinized by others. The most well-known and efficacious psychological treatment for individuals with SAD is cognitive behavior therapy (CBT). Previous meta-analysis reported that the most recommended treatment components of CBT programs for SAD are exposure and cognitive restructuring. In recent years, mindfulness-based intervention (MBI) has shown efficacy in improving SAD. In this chapter, exposure treatment and cognitive restructuring for SAD and MBI for SAD are introduced. Additionally, the benefits of using MBI for SAD are discussed. This chapter also discusses the effects on the improvement of trait-mindfulness for social anxiety. Finally, we indicate the possibilities of the combination of mindfulness and exposure for treatment of SAD.

Keywords: social anxiety disorder, cognitive behavior therapy, exposure treatment, mindfulness

1. Introduction

Social anxiety disorder (SAD) is the most common anxiety disorder and is characterized by a fear of negative evaluation by others [1, 2]. Patients with SAD or high socially anxious individuals perceive high anxiety in social situations and often avoid social situations. SAD impairs the social, academic, occupational, and economic functioning of patients [3]. SAD is one of the most prevalent mental disorders. Its prevalence in the community is indicated as being up to 13% [4]. The other epidemiological literature reports that its lifetime prevalence in Western countries ranges between 7% and 12% [5, 6]. In Japanese samples [7] from the World Mental Health Japan (WMHJ) survey, researchers estimated that the 12 month prevalence of SAD was 0.8% among Japanese people. This face-to-face household survey involved 1663 adults (overall response rate, 56%) in four communities in Japan, including two cities and two rural population areas. It is also suggested that there is a continuum between social anxieties or fears and SAD.

Individuals with SAD are often afraid of social situations and social interaction. For example, these situations are public speaking, conversation, telephone, writing, and so on. Individuals, who have excessive fear of public speaking, often avoid this activity because they have various negative cognitive assumptions and images about failure to give an "adequate" performance. Before a speaking session, they feel too much anxiety and perceive physical arousal symptoms. In addition, they think that they will not deliver a good performance and that catastrophic things will happen. When conducting their tasks, they feel that they cannot control outcomes and their performance. They do not look at the faces in their audience and they speak fast. Afterwards they realize that their speech was bad and they will be evaluated as "negative" or "insignificant" people. Therefore, they usually avoid these situations.

These negative cognition and avoidance behaviors are traditionally summarized in a cognitive model or cognitive behavior model. In this chapter, we report on the previous cognitive behavior therapy (CBT) model of SAD and the technique of CBT for SAD. Additionally, we introduce recent research in mindfulness-based therapy and discuss the future direction of a psychotherapy that takes SAD into account.

1.1. The cognitive behavior therapy model

Cognitive and cognitive-behavioral models of SAD posit that negative cognition maintains social anxiety symptoms. These models describe the relationships between negative cognition, behavior, and somatic symptoms in SAD. In these models, cognition includes self-focused attention, interpretation, rumination, self-perception, social negative evaluation, and other cognitive values [8, 9]. Clark and Wells [8] suggested that patients with SAD develop a series of negative assumptions and overestimate how negatively other people will evaluate their performance in social situations. In social situations, patients with SAD perceive social danger for themselves. These negative processing biases produce somatic symptoms and behavioral symptoms, which interact to heighten social anxiety symptoms. In their cognitive-behavioral model, Rapee and Heimberg [9] suggested that individuals with SAD and highly socially anxious individuals have a greater expectancy of negative occurrences. Also, they predict a greater cost of these occurrences for themselves than do less anxious individuals in social situations. Additionally, they indicated that these probability and cost estimates are related to state anxiety in social situations.

The estimated social cost of this is a specific expression of dysfunctional beliefs about the potential outcome of a social encounter [10]. The cognitive behavioral model of Hofmann and Otto provided general treatment model of SAD. In the model, maintaining the factors of SAD is discussed and indicates the importance of the overestimation of the negative consequences, the perception of low emotional control, negative self-perceptions, negative rumination, and so on. Symptoms of SAD can be classified into cognitive, behavioral, and physical categories [11]. Cognitive symptoms include negative self-evaluations or catastrophizing what other people think of the individual in social situations. Individuals with SAD may have thoughts such as

"I am stupid," "Everyone thinks I'm acting weird," and so on. People with SAD tend to think that their thoughts are factual and put too much focus on them. Behavioral symptoms include avoiding or prematurely escaping from social situations to reduce anxiety or avoid negative evaluation by others. Individuals who cannot avoid or escape may engage in safety behaviors [12].

1.2. Cognitive behavior therapy: CBT for SAD

There are several studies of effective treatment for SAD [13–17]. These treatment programs include psycho-education, exposure, cognitive restructuring, and original interventions. Typical CBT techniques for the treatment of SAD include exposure, applied relaxation, social skills training, and cognitive restructuring [17]. In their meta-analytic review, they reported that the most recommended treatment components of CBT programs are exposure and cognitive restructuring. Clark et al. [18] reported high-effect levels for individual CBT. This program consisted of helping clients to develop a list of personal safety behaviors, conducting self-focused attention experiments where the focus of attention is shifted to social situations, psychoeducation about their model [8], video feedback, behavioral experiments, identification of problematic anticipatory and post-event processing, and modification of assumptions about dysfunction. Depending on the assessment point, uncontrolled effect levels in their study ranged from 2.14 to 2.53.

Rapee et al. [14] examined possible differences between standard cognitive behavioral group therapy (CBGT) and an enhanced CBGT program. Standard CBGT consisted of standard cognitive restructuring plus in vivo exposure. The enhanced CBGT program was augmented with several additional treatment techniques, including performance feedback and attention retraining. These programs were conducted in therapist facilitated groups of approximately six participants. Both types of CBGT package had sufficient improvement on SAD symptoms, with the enhanced treatment showing better effects than standard treatment on the cost of negative evaluation and negative views of one's skills and appearance.

CBT for SAD is classified as both group therapy and individual therapy. Both types of therapies have merits and demerits as discussed in the following section. The merits of group therapy are: (1) presence of others when being exposed in social conditions is useful for increasing the degree of a threat and reality; (2) others' modeling becomes possible in exposure settings; (3) cooperative consciousness among patients toward treatment is developed; and (4) simultaneous intervention for various patients become possible, among others. On the other hand, group therapy has some demerits as follows: (1) presence of others might activate fears of negative evaluation, which might inhibit patients' spontaneous behaviors and speeches; (2) the threat of exposure might increase excessively; (3) the relationships between therapists and patients tend to become weak; and (4) the presence of others might make it difficult for participants to participate in the program, among other problems. The merits of individual therapies are: (1) therapists can easily adapt the program to the cognitive and behavior characteristics of each patient; (2) participation in treatment is easier, compared to group therapy; (3) individual patients' needs and questions are sufficiently dealt with; and (4) participants can freely express their speeches and behaviors without considering others, among other benefits. On the other hand, it is considered difficult to get the merits of group therapy as described earlier through individual therapies, from the perspective of its structure.

1.3. Exposure

Exposure technique is one of the best ways to deal with SAD symptoms. In the treatment of SAD, in vivo exposure often has been used. In exposure therapy, the following approaches are involved: psychological education about exposure, development of anxiety hierarchy worksheets, specifying exposure settings, execution of exposure, and anxiety assessment before and after exposure. In psychological education, participants learn in advance the characteristics of anxiety and what will be conducted in exposure therapy. They need to sufficiently understand the nature of psychological burden when implementing the therapy.

Through developing an anxiety hierarchy worksheet, the situation of anxiety and the degree of anxiety in each situation become clear. Through setting discussion in concrete situations, problems are shared between the therapist and client. The first aim of exposure therapy is to reduce anxiety. Social settings tend to change in the condition where anxiety feelings are high. For example, speech situations usually finish in a few minutes. Participants tend to finish the situation with high anxiety, which leads to avoidance behaviors in the next anxiety situation. It is important to properly expose themselves to each anxiety situation repeatedly. Exposure therapy is often conducted during a treatment session (regardless of inside or outside of the treatment institutions) or in an actual setting as homework. Though imagined exposure is also effective, when exposure in real life can be used, this can be related to daily situations.

1.4. Cognitive biases

There are some types of information-processing biases in SAD. Attentional biases, interpretation biases, memory biases, and cost/probability biases are often modified in bias modification. The effects of cognitive restructuring have been indicated through various studies. For example, Clark et al. [19] indicated the following as intervention targets of cognitive therapy: (1) attention, or an increase in attention and reduction in observation of others and making association with others' responses; (2) recognition of physiological responses, or the use of incorrect inner information that causes excessively negative ideas about how others think of the self; (3) safety behaviors (avoidance), or the excessive use of explicit or implicit safety behaviors; and (4): information-processing biases, or the processing of information before and after an issue. They thus compared the effects of cognitive therapy and exposure + applied relaxation therapy. The results indicated the high impact of cognitive therapy on improving SAD symptoms, indicative of the effectiveness of the intervention in cognition characteristic of SAD.

The research on the treatment of SAD has thus focused on the effectiveness of using cognitive therapy techniques to change specific cognitions or thought patterns [14, 18, 19]. However, SAD treatment research has also focused on the reduction of cost and probability bias. Foa et al. [20] reported that the reduction of cost bias strongly predicted the reduction of SAD symptoms. Rapee et al. [14] showed that a change in cost bias was highly related to a decrease in the severity of SAD symptoms using a group CBT (CBGT) program. Shirotsuki et al. [21] suggested that repeated exposure and reduction of cost bias may have an effect on the improvement of SAD symptoms.

1.5. Video feedback

Video feedback (VF) is one of the important and effective techniques in most CBT treatment programs. Individuals with SAD try to watch their video before receiving sufficient cognitive preparation. Clark et al. [18] reported a high impact from individual CBT. This program consisted of developing with patients a personal set of safety behaviors and a self-focused attention experiment: shifting the focus of attention to the social situation. In video feedback sessions, individuals with SAD watch their actual social tasks, which are public speaking and conversation. They often recognize their performance is worse than actual performance. Therapists try to change the discrepancy between subjective and objective perceptions of social performance. VF involves providing individuals with video playback of their social performance following their participation about social task, such as a public speech or a one-on-one conversation [22]. High socially anxious and individuals with SAD watch the real situation through recorded video. Video feedback involves video recording socially anxious individuals while they are trying a social task, that is, a speaking task or conversation. It is anticipated that review of the recording corrects distorted self-evaluations, including the underestimation of social skills [23].

Though video feedback sessions are effective, it is necessary to consider that participants might have a resulting psychological burden. Shirotsuki [24] indicated the effects of the interpretation of video images: when watching video images, sometimes, participants cannot perceive themselves objectively owing to their negative interpretation of the video images, which reduces the self-evaluation of their performance. It is considered important to try to make participants watch video images objectively before the session.

1.6. Mindfulness

In recent years, researchers and clinicians have developed intervention programs that include mindfulness. Mindfulness is defined as "paying attention in a particular way—on purpose, in the present moment and nonjudgmentally" [25]. Bishop et al. [26] distinguished two components of mindfulness. The first component is "self-regulation of attention." Self-regulation of attention is observing and attending to the changing field of thoughts, feeling, and sensations from moment to moment. This leads to a feeling of being very alert to what is occurring in the here-and-now [26].

The second component is "orientation to experience." Orientation to experience is an attitude of openness, acceptance, and curiosity about the present moment. Experiential avoidance which is the opposite concept of orientation to experience is at the heart of all psychological distress [27]. It is to avoid one's own experience such as thought, feeling, cognition, behavior, and sense of body. Experiential avoidance is reduced by increasing the mental state of orientation to experience; as a result, psychological distress improves [28].

Many researchers have found relationship between trait mindfulness and mental health criteria. Baer et al. showed that trait mindfulness was negatively correlated with alexithymia, dissociative activities, difficulties in emotion regulation, and neuroticism [29]. Higher levels of trait mindfulness predict lower levels of anxiety, depression, and negative cognition, and higher levels of well-being [30]. Coffey et al. found that the improvement of trait mindfulness has been found to positively influence mental health [31]. The improvement of trait mindfulness also negatively impacts on anxiety, depression, and negative cognition [31, 32]. To enhance levels of trait mindfulness, mindfulness training (MT) can be used. MT includes body scan, gentle mindful yoga exercises, sitting meditation, walking meditation, eating meditation, among others (**Table 1**). MT is effective for improving stress, stress reactivity, anxiety, and depression [30, 33–35].

1.7. The relationship between trait mindfulness and social anxiety

Some researchers have started to examine the effects of mindfulness on social anxiety. Previous studies have reported that trait mindfulness is negatively correlated with self-reported social anxiety, and trait mindfulness has a direct effect on social anxiety [36, 37]. Kocovski et al. also indicated that trait mindfulness predicts subsequent changes in social anxiety and that social anxiety predicts subsequent change in trait mindfulness [38]. Recent studies have provided relationships among trait mindfulness, social anxiety, and maintaining factors of social anxiety as mechanism of mindfulness on social anxiety. According to Clark and Wells and Rapee and Heimberg [8, 9], self-regulation of attention, avoidance behavior, and negative cognition are the factors that maintain SAD social anxiety disorder (SAD).

Noda et al. showed that trait mindfulness affects social anxiety through self-regulation of attention, avoidance behavior, and fear of negative evaluation by others in negative cognition,

Techniques	Features
Body scan	The aim is to be aware of the sensation of your body you pay attention to, and accept nonjudgmentally occuring experience at the time. You can monitor the sensation of body in here and now. You can also improve sensitivity of body.
Gentle mindful yoga exercises	The aim is to be aware of what is experiencing in your body while doing yoga.You can monitor one's present monent experience, in here and now, such as stretching. You can experience "myself as a whole".
Sitting meditation	The aim is to pay attention to breath, be aware of the flow of breathing. By paying attention to breathing, you can focus on here and now. And you be aware the sensation of body that accompanies breathing.
Walking meditation	The aim is to be aware of something you are experiencing while walking.You can be aware the sensation of the foot, the sensation of the body accompanied with walking, the sensation with the ground. You can be aware of "sense of your presence in the place".
Eating meditation	The aim is to be aware of the sensations of smelling, tasting, chewing, and swallowing through eating. You can monitor the five senses in here and now.

Table 1. Main techniques and simple features of mindfulness training.

while Schmertz et al. reported that trait mindfulness impacts on social anxiety via cost/probability bias in negative cognition [37, 39]. Moreover, Okawa et al. showed that trait mindfulness affects social anxiety via rumination in negative cognition [40]. **Figure 1**, based on the earlier research, provides a mechanism for assessing the impact of mindfulness on social anxiety. This indicates that trait mindfulness affects social anxiety through maintaining various factors. Based on this research, it is considered that an increase in trait mindfulness would be not only effective for social anxiety but also for its maintenance factors. Research such as this supports the conclusion that trait mindfulness is strongly related to social anxiety symptoms.

Additional treatment studies of MT for SAD patients have been conducted. Previous research has reported that MT is effective in treating social anxiety symptoms [41, 42]. A therapeutic intervention program that includes MT is called Mindfulness-Based Intervention (MBI). MBI for SAD includes Mindfulness-Based Stress Reduction (MBSR), Mindfulness-Based Cognitive Therapy (MBCT), Acceptance and Commitment Therapy (ACT), and Mindfulness and Acceptance-based Group Therapy (MAGT).

1.8. Mindfulness-based stress reduction

MBSR was developed by Kabat-Zinn [43]. It is the most well-known MBI and has gained empirical support in the treatment of psychological symptoms. The protocol of MBSR is composed of MT. Previous research has shown that MBSR is effective for treating stress, anxiety, depression symptoms, improving self-regulation, and the purpose of life [34, 44]. Goldin and Gross [41] conducted MBSR for SAD patients. Individuals (N = 16) diagnosed with SAD participated in 8 weekly 2.5 h sessions of MBSR. The main components of treatment were mindfulness meditation techniques such as breath-focused attention, body scan-based attention to the transient nature of sensory experience, shifting attention across sensory modalities, open

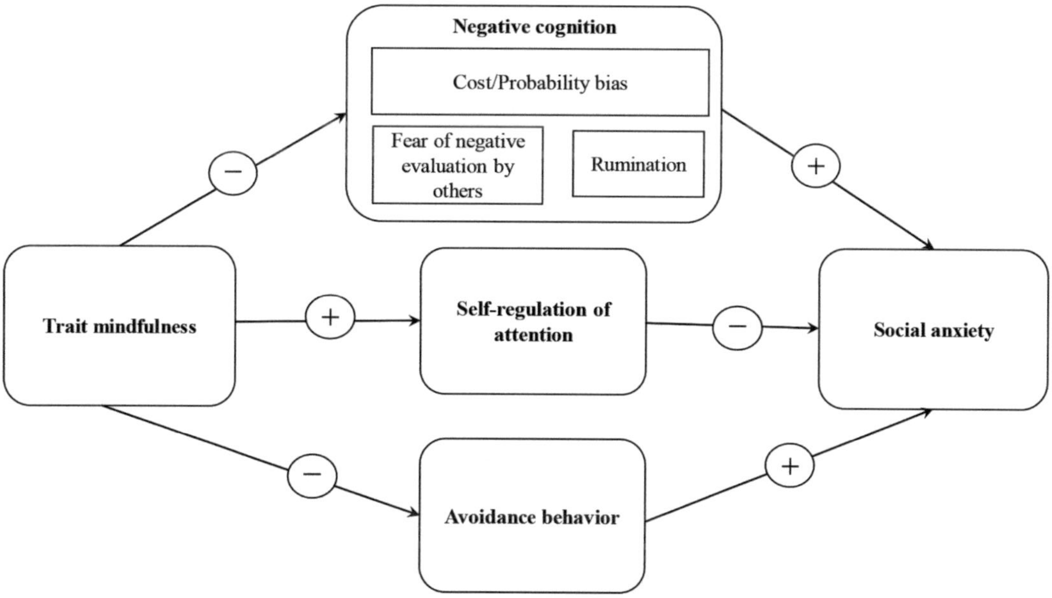

Figure 1. The mechanism of mindfulness on social anxiety.

monitoring of moment-to-moment experience, walking meditation, and eating meditation. As a result, MBSR showed significant reduction in self-reported social anxiety symptoms and negative cognition ($\eta^2p = .59$ on the Liebowitz Social Anxiety Scale; $\eta^2p = .53$ on the Rumination Style Questionnaire) and significant improvement in self-reported self-esteem ($\eta^2p = .51$ on the Rosenberg Self-Esteem Scale). In another study, individuals (N = 22) diagnosed with SAD participated in 8 weekly 2.5 h sessions of MBSR and an all-day meditation retreat for MBSR [42]. The MBSR produced significant reductions in self-reported social anxiety symptoms effect size (ES) = 1.48 on the Liebowitz Social Anxiety Scale-Fear; ES = 1.40 on the Liebowitz Social Anxiety Scale-Avoidance).

1.9. Mindfulness-based cognitive therapy

MBCT is developed to prevent relapse of major depression [45]. It combines elements of cognitive therapy approach and MT to reduce the symptoms of depression and the recurrence of depression. Teasdale et al. [46] found MBCT has prevented relapse and recurrence in patients with a history of three or more episodes of depression. MBCT is not only effective for depression but also other disorders. Piet et al. [47] conducted MBSR for SAD patients. Fourteen young participants aged 18–25 years with SAD participated in 8 weekly 2 h sessions of MBCT. The main components of treatment were mindfulness meditation techniques such as body scans, gentle mindful yoga exercises, and sitting meditation. The result of this intervention study showed that the MBCT produced significant prepost improvements with moderate to high ESs (0.77 on the Social Phobia Composite measure, and 0.90 on the Liebowitz Social Anxiety Scale).

1.10. Acceptance and commitment therapy

The theoretical basis of ACT is a relational frame construct that is a behavior analytic theory of language and cognition [27]. It focuses on understanding behavior through linguistic contexts or frames. It also includes techniques designed to promote mindful awareness of internal experiences. ACT aims to promote namely the improvement of orientation to experience and cognitive defusing that is a shifting of mental contexts by cultivating patient's awareness of awareness to allow them to view thoughts as thoughts and not as facts [27, 28]. Dalrymple and Herbert [48] conducted ACT for SAD patients. Nineteen individuals diagnosed with SAD participated in a 12 weekly 1 h program integrating exposure therapy and ACT. The results revealed that significant improvements occurred in self-reported social anxiety symptoms, yielding large effect size gains (ES = 0.72 on the Liebowitz Social Anxiety Scale-Fear, ES = 1.24 on the Liebowitz Social Anxiety Scale-Avoidance). In another study by Ossman et al. [49], individuals (N = 22) diagnosed with SAD participated in 10 weekly 2 h sessions of ACT. Here, ACT produced significant reductions in self-reported social anxiety symptoms (ES = 0.82 on the Liebowitz Social Anxiety Scale-Fear and ES = 1.71 on the Liebowitz Social Anxiety Scale-Avoidance).

1.11. Mindfulness and acceptance-based group therapy

The MAGT for SAD developed by Fleming and Kocovski [50] was based on the ACT. Some of the mindfulness exercises included in this protocol could be adapted from the MBCT. The main components of treatment in the protocol are mindfulness exercises, and acceptance of thoughts and feelings, and acceptance of social anxiety exercises. Kocovski et al. conducted MAGT for SAD patients [51]. Individuals (N = 53) diagnosed with SAD participated in 12 weekly 2 h sessions of MAGT. Consequently, the MAGT results showed significant reductions in self-reported social anxiety symptoms (d = 1.32 on the Social Phobia Inventory). In another study [52], individuals (N = 29) diagnosed with SAD participated in 12 weekly 2 h sessions of MAGT. As a result, the MAGT produced significant prepost improvements with high ESs (1.00 on the Liebowitz Social Anxiety Scale, 1.09 on the Social Phobia Scale, and 1.03 on the Social Interaction Anxiety Scale). From the earlier research, MBI appears to be an effective intervention for SAD, with generally large effect sizes on social anxiety symptoms.

2. Future direction

2.1. The possibilities in the combination of mindfulness and exposure for the treatment of SAD

The most well-known and effective psychological treatment for individuals with SAD is cognitive behavioral therapy (CBT). However, although CBT has been found to be efficacious in reducing social anxiety, there are patients who do not achieve clinically significant improvement following CBT [17]. According to Leichsenring et al., remission rates were nearly 40% for CBT [53]. Thus, the development of intervention protocols that are more effective for improving social anxiety symptoms than traditional CBT is demanded.

Exposure, which is a key ingredient of most CBT, is effective for improving social anxiety symptoms [54]. But, it is indicated that exposure tend to be avoided and dropped by patients [55]. According to Van Velzen et al., 34.4% of patients with SAD dropped-out from exposure programs [56]. In another study by Hofmann, the attrition rate of exposure group therapy was 21% [23]. From the above, it is considered that exposure is an intervention that carries with a strong mental burden.

The crucial factor causing patients with SAD to avoid and drop-out from exposure is experiential avoidance, which is based on thoughts, feelings, cognition, behavior, and sensation in the body in social situations. Experiential avoidance is a disturbance factor in the effective treatment of exposure, promoting the maintenance of anxiety [55]. By enhancing mental state of mindfulness, we would be promoted to increase awareness of one's experience and to accept what we are currently experiencing. Thereby, experiential avoidance is reduced [44], and willingness enhanced [55]. These findings suggest that incorporating MT into exposure for treatment of SAD may prevent patients from avoiding and dropping-out exposure. The combination of cognitive approach and exposure is thus more effective for improving social anxiety symptoms than only exposure [54]. Because MT seeks to reduce negative cognition [41, 47], and to enhance decentering and change cognitive flexibility [44], it functions as an approach that changes negative cognition. In addition, MT brings the improvement of self-regulation to our attention [41]. The low self-regulation of attention is core maintaining factors of social anxiety [8]. These findings suggest that the combination of MT and exposure may be more effective for improving social anxiety symptoms than traditional exposure therapy.

We propose the following procedure as the most appropriate combination of mindfulness and exposure for SAD. First, MT is conducted. Through MT patients will be persuaded to increase their awareness of experiences such as negative cognition, social anxiety, trembling, and sweating in social situation, and then it leads to accept these experiences. As a result, negative cognition, social anxiety, and fear of physical response are alleviated. The effect of maintaining factors on social anxiety would be reduced. Therefore, the mental burden of patients to exposure would reduce, and these effects may prevent patients from avoiding and dropping-out exposure. In addition, maintaining mechanism of social anxiety would improve. This shows that MT could prevent relapse and recurrence following therapy.

Second, exposure is reinforced. Through exposure the therapist encourages patients to face anxiety in social situations. They should notice their experience in facing social situations. And they may understand the differences in their experience between preexposure and post-exposure situations. Exposure thus produces a significant reduction in social anxiety [54]. Because social anxiety would be improved by MT, exposure after MT may be more effective for improving social anxiety and maintaining the effect of treatment than exposure alone.

Acknowledgements

This study was supported by Grant-in-Aid for Scientific Research (C) "KAKENHI" Number 17 K04463.

Author details

Kentaro Shirotsuki[1]* and Shota Noda[2]

*Address all correspondence to: kenshiro@musashino-u.ac.jp

1 Faculty of Human Sciences, Musashino University, Tokyo, Japan

2 Graduate School of Human and Social Sciences, Musashino University, Tokyo, Japan

References

[1] American Psychiatric Association. Diagnostic and Statistical Manual of Mental Disorders. 4th ed. Washington, DC: American Psychiatric Association; 1994

[2] Kessler RC, McGonagle UA, Zhao S, Nelson CB, Hughes M, Eshleman S, Wittchen H, Kendler KS. Life-time and 12-month prevalence of DSM-III-R psychiatric disorders in the United States. Archives of General Psychiatry. 1994;**51**:8-19

[3] Katzelnick DJ, Greist JH. Social anxiety disorder: An unrecognized problem in primary care. The Journal of Clinical Psychiatry. 2001;**62**:11-15

[4] Ruscio AM, Brown TA, Chiu WT, Sareen J, Stein MB, Kessler RC. Social fears and social phobia in the United States: Results from the National Comorbidity Survey Replication. Psychological Medicine. 2008;**38**:15-28

[5] Furmark T. Social phobia: Overview of community surveys. Acta Psychiatrica Scandinavica. 2002;**105**:84-93. DOI: 10.1034/j.1600-0447.2002.1r103.x

[6] Kessler RC, Berglund PD, Demler O, Olga JR, Merikangas KR, Walters EE. Lifetime prevalence and age-of-onset distributions of DSM-IV disorders in the National Comorbidity Survey replication. Archives of General Psychiatry. 2005;**62**:593-602

[7] Kawakami N, Takeshima T, Ono Y, Uda H, Hata Y, Nakane Y, et al. Twelve-month prevalence, severity, and treatment of common mental disorders in communities in Japan: A preliminary finding from the world mental health Japan survey 2002-2003. Psychiatry and Clinical Neurosciences. 2005;**59**:441-452. DOI: 10.1111/j.1440-1819.2005.01397

[8] Clark DM, Wells AA. Cognitive model of social phobia. In: Heimberg RG, Liebowitz MR, Hope DA, Schneier FR, editors. Social Phobia: Diagnosis, Assessment, and Treatment. New York: Guilford Press; 1995. pp. 69-93

[9] Rapee RM, Heimberg RG. A cognitive-behavioral model of anxiety in social phobia. Behavior Research and Therapy. 1997;**35**:741-756

[10] Hofmann SG, Otto MW. Cognitive Behavior Therapy for Social Anxiety Disorder: Evidence-Based and Disorder-Specific Treatment Techniques (Practical Guidebooks Series). New York: Routledge; 2008

[11] Heimberg RG, Brozovich FA, Rapee RM. A cognitive-behavioral model of social anxiety disorder: Update and extension. In: Hofmann SG, DiBartolo PM, editors. Social Anxiety: Clinical, Developmental and Social Perspectives. New York: Elsevier; 2010. pp. 395-422

[12] Piccirillo ML, Dryman MT, Heimberg RG. Safety behaviors in adults with social anxiety: Review and future directions. Behavior Therapy. 2016;**47**:675-687

[13] Hofmann SG. Cognitive factors that maintain social anxiety disorder: A comprehensive model and its treatment implications. Cognitive Behaviour Therapy. 2007;**36**(4):193-209

[14] Rapee RM, Gaston JE, Abbott MJ. Testing the efficacy of theoretically derived improvements in the treatment of social phobia. Journal of Consulting and Clinical Psychology. 2009;**77**:317-327. DOI: 10.1037/a0014800

[15] Heimberg RG, Salzman DG, Holt CS, Blendell KA. Cognitive-behavioral group treatment for social phobia: Effectiveness at five-year follow-up. Cognitive Therapy and Research. 1993;**17**:325-339

[16] Heimberg RG. Cognitive-behavioral therapy for social anxiety disorder: Current status and future directions. Biological Psychiatry. 2002;**51**:101-108. DOI: 10.1016/S0006-3223(01)01183-0

[17] Rodebaugh TL, Holaway RM, Heimberg RG. The treatment of social anxiety disorder. Clinical Psychological Review. 2004;**24**:883-908. DOI: 10.1016/j.cpr.2004.07.007

[18] Clark DM, Ehlers A, McManus F, Hackmann A, Fennell M, Campbell H, et al. Cognitive therapy versus fluoxetine in generalized social phobia: A randomized placebo-controlled trial. Journal of Consulting and Clinical Psychology. 2003;**7**:1058-1067

[19] Clark DM, Ehlers A, Hackmann A, McManus F, Fennell M, Grey N, et al. Cognitive therapy versus exposure and applied relaxation in social phobia: A randomized controlled trial. Journal of Consulting and Clinical Psychology. 2006;**74**:568-578. DOI: 10.1037/0022-006X.74.3.568

[20] Foa EB, Franklin ME, Perry KJ, Herbert JD. Cognitive biases in social phobia. Journal of Abnormal Psychology. 1996;**105**:433-439. DOI: 10.1037/0021-843X.105.3.433

[21] Shirotsuki K, Kodama Y, Nomura S. The preliminary study of individual cognitive behavior therapy for Japanese patients with social anxiety disorder. Psychological Services. 2014;**11**:162-170

[22] Orr EMJ, Moscovitch DA. Learning to re-appraise the self during video feedback for social anxiety: Does depth of processing matter? Behaviour Research and Therapy. 2010;**48**: 728-737

[23] Hofmann SG. Cognitive mediation of treatment change in social phobia. Journal of Consulting and Clinical Psychology. 2004;**72**:392-399

[24] Shirotsuki K. Negative and positive interpretations of appearance on video in socially-anxious individuals. Bulletin of the Clinical Psychology Center, Musashino University. 2013;**13**:1-9

[25] Kabat-Zinn J. Wherever you Go, there you Are : Mindfulness Meditation in Everyday Life. New York: Hyperion; 1994

[26] Bishop SR, Lau M, Shapiro S, Carlson L, Anderson ND, Carmody J, Devins G. Mindfulness: A proposed operational definition. Clinical Psychology: Science and Practice. 2004;**11**:230-241

[27] Annunziata AJ, Green JD, Marx BP. Acceptance and commitment therapy for depression and anxiety. In: Friedman HS, editor. Encyclopedia of Mental Health. 2nd ed. New York: Academic Press; 2015. pp. 1-10

[28] Bach PA, Moran DJ. ACT in Practice: Case Conceptualization in Acceptance & Commitment Therapy. Oakland: New Harbinger Publications; 2008

[29] Baer RA, Smith GT, Hopkins J, Krietemeyer J, Toney L. Using self-report assessment methods to explore facets of mindfulness. Assessment. 2006;**13**:27-45

[30] Brown KW, Ryan RM. The benefits of being present: Mindfulness and its role in psychological well-being. Journal of Personality and Social Psychology. 2003;**84**:822-848

[31] Coffey KA, Hartman M, Fredrickson BL. Deconstructing mindfulness and constructing mental health: Understanding mindfulness and its mechanisms. Mindfulness. 2010;**1**: 235-253

[32] Bajaj B, Robins WR, Pande N. Mediating role of self-esteem on the relationship between mindfulness, anxiety, and depression. Personality and Individual Differences. 2016;**96**: 127-131

[33] Creswell JD, Pacilio LE, Lindsay EK, Brown KW. Brief mindfulness mediation training alters psychological and neuroendocrine responses to social evaluative stress. Psychoneuro. 2014;**44**:1-12

[34] Kabat-Zinn J, Massion AO, Kristeller J, Peterson LG, Fletcher KE, Pbert L, Lenderking WR, Santorelli SF. Effectiveness of a meditation-based stress reduction program in the treatment of anxiety disorder. The American Journal of Psychiatry. 1992;**149**:936-943

[35] Kumar SM, Feldman GC, Hayes AM. Changes in mindfulness and emotion regulation in an exposure-based cognitive therapy for depression. Cognitive Therapy and Research. 2008;**32**:734-744

[36] Rasmussen MK, Pidgeon AM. The direct and indirect benefits of dispositional mindfulness on self-esteem and social anxiety. Anxiety, Stress, and Coping. 2011;**24**:227-233

[37] Schmertz SK, Masuda A, Anderson PL. Cognitive processes mediate the relation between mindfulness and social anxiety within a clinical sample. Journal of Clinical Psychology. 2012;**68**:362-371

[38] Kocovski NL, Fleming JE, Hawley LL, Ho MR, Antony MM. Mindfulness and acceptance-based group therapy and traditional cognitive behavioral group therapy for social anxiety disorder: Mechanisms of change. Behaviour Resarch and Therapy. 2015;**70**:11-22

[39] Noda S, Okawa S, Shirotsuki K. The relationship among the trait mindfulness, self-regulation of attention, fear of negative evaluation, avoidance behavior, and social anxiety. Japanese Association of Mindfulness. 2017;**2**:11-21

[40] Okawa S, Noda S, Shirotsuki K. The relationship among the trait mindfulness, depression symptoms, social anxiety, the maintaining factors. The 17th Annual Meeting of the Japanese Association for Cognitive Therapy. Tokyo, July 22; 2017

[41] Goldin PR, Gross JJ. Effects of mindfulness-based stress reduction (MBSR) on emotion regulation in social anxiety disorder. Emotion. 2010;**10**:83-91

[42] Koszycki D, Benger M, Shlik J, Bradwejn J. Randomized trial of a meditation-based stress reduction program and cognitive behavbior therapy in generalized social anxiety disorder. Behaviour Research and Therapy. 2007;**45**:2518-2526

[43] Kabat-Zinn J. An outpatient program in behavioral medicine for chronic pain patients based on the practice of mindfulness meditation: Theoretical considerations and preliminary results. General Hospital Psychiatry. 1982;**4**:33-47

[44] Carmody J, Baer RA, Lykins ELB, Olendzki N. An empirical study of the mechanisms of mindfulness in a mindfulness-based stress reduction program. Journal of Clinical Psychology. 2009;**65**:613-626

[45] Segal ZV, Williams JM, Teasdale J. Mindfulness-Based Cognitive Therapy for Depression. New York: Guilford Press; 2002

[46] Teasdale JD, Segal ZV, Williams JM, Ridgeway VA, Soulsby JM, Lau MA. Prevention of relapse/recurrence in major depression by mindfulness-based cognitive therapy. Journal of Consulting and Clinical Psychology. 2000;**68**:615-623

[47] Piet J, Hougaard E, Hecksher MS, Rosenberg NK. A randomized pilot study of mindfulness-based cognitive therapy and group cognitive-behavioral therapy for young adults with social phobia. Scandinavian Journal of Psychology. 2010;**51**:403-410

[48] Dalrymple KL, Herbert JD. Acceptance and commitment therapy for generalized social anxiety disorder: A pilot study. Behavior Modification. 2007;**31**:543-568

[49] Ossman WA, Wilson KG, Storaashi RD, McNeill JW. Apreliminary investigation of the use of acceptance and commitment therapy in group treatment for social phobia. International Journal of Psychology and Psychological Therapy. 2006;**6**:397-416

[50] Fleming JE, Kocovski NL. Mindfulness and acceptance-based group therapy for social anxiety disorder: A treatment manual. Unpublished manuscript; 2007. Retrieved from www.actonsocialanxiety.com/pdf/Treatment_Manual.pdf

[51] Kocovski NL, Fleming JE, Hawley LL, Huta V, Antony MM. Mindfulness and acceptance-based group therapy versus traditional cognitive behavioral group therapy for social anxiety disorder: A randomized controlled trial. Behaviour Research and Therapy. 2013;**51**:889-898

[52] Kocovski NL, Fleming JE, Rector NA. Mindfulness and acceptance-based group therapy for social anxiety disorder: An open trial. Cognitive and Behavioral Practice. 2009;**16**:276-289

[53] Leichsenring F, Salzer S, Beutel ME, Herpertz S, Hiller W, Hoyer J, Huesing J, Joraschky P, Nolting B, Poehlman K, Ritter V, Stangier U, Strauss B, Tefikow H, Teismann T, Willutzki U, Wiltink J, Leibing E. Long-term outcome of psychodynamic therapy and cognitive-behavioral therapy in social anxiety disorder. The American Journal of Psychiatry. 2014;**171**: 1074-1082

[54] Mattick RP, Peters L, Clarkc JC. Exposure and cognitive restructuring for social phobia: A controlled study. Behavior Therapy. 1989;**20**:3-23

[55] Sisemore TA. The clinician's Guide to Exposure Therapies for Anxiety Spectrum Disorder: Integrating Techniques and Applications from CBT, DBT, and ACT. Oakland: New Harbinger Publications; 2012

[56] Van Velzen CJM, Emmelkamp PMG, Scholing A. The impact of personality disorders on behavioural treatment outcome for social phobia. Behaviour Research and Therapy. 1997;**35**:889-900